Backache

WHAT EXERCISES *REALLY* WORK

Also by Dava Sobel and Arthur C. Klein

Arthritis: What Really Works
Arthritis: What Exercises Really Work

Backache

WHAT EXERCISES *REALLY* WORK

Dava Sobel &
Arthur C. Klein

Robinson
LONDON

Robinson Publishing Ltd
7 Kensington Church Court
London W8 4SP

First published in the UK by Robinson Publishing Ltd 1996

Collection © Dava Sobel and Arthur C. Klein 1994
Illustrations by Lauren Jarrett

Important Note
This book is not intended to be a substitute for medical advice or
treatment. Any person with a condition requiring medical
attention should consult a qualified medical practitioner or
suitable therapist.

A copy of the British Library Cataloguing in Publication data
is available from the British Library

ISBN 1-85487-491-8

Printed and bound in the EC

10 9 8 7 6 5 4 3 2

CONTENTS

FOREWORD TO THE UK EDITION

Back pain is much the commonest of all chronic ailments because there are more muscles, nerves, bones, joints and ligaments running up the length of the spine in close proximity to each other than in any other part of the body. Further, as the chronic back pain sufferer soon realizes, this subtle complexity of spinal structures is such that for the vast majority even the best trained doctors with the most sophisticated of diagnostic equipment are unable to determine the precise source of their misfortune.

Thus the best protection against back problems is to maintain the strength and suppleness of the spine by regular exercises, and yet in dozens of articles I have read over the years on this subject, hardly ever is this point emphasized.

Dava Sobel and Arthur Klein have finally corrected this omission in a book that draws on the richest and most diverse source of all therapeutic wisdom – people's own experience. Indeed one of the main problems about back pain is that we have come to rely too heavily on the views and opinions of experts, which anyhow go in and out of fashion. In their pioneering book *Arthritis – What Really Works*, the authors canvassed thousands of sufferers to produce the best popular guide that had ever been written on the subject. They repeated this winning formula interviewing 500 back pain sufferers for their book *Backache Relief*, which convincingly showed that a therapeutic programme offered the greatest help.

Here they describe lucidly and sympathetically the precise details of such an exercise programme which has been judged safe and effective by specialists at the New York hospital, Cornell University Medical Centre.

Like all family doctors, I see on average a couple of patients with back pain every week and am delighted that in addition to other appropriate advice and specialist referral I can now recommend a book that offers the best hope of long-term cure for many of them.

—Dr James Le Fanu

PART
ONE

The Magic Bullet

> There is indeed a "magic bullet"
> that can effectively cure back pain.
> It is called exercise, and it works.

A NOTE FOR THE UK EDITION

Throughout the book, some terms common to the US rather than the UK are used. Your physical therapist means your physiotherapist, and orthopedist is an orthopaedic surgeon, for example. The term physiatrist does not have an exact equivalent in the UK, the closest probably being a physician who specializes in rehabilitation. In addition, the symbol # is sometimes used to indicate 'number'. There are also references to private health care costs which do not apply to the UK in the same way.

Many of the exercises in this book involve getting on to the floor. To help you get down to this position, we advise you to: drop down on to your hands and knees; then roll on to one side by first lowering your bottom, then your shoulders, to the floor. You can then roll on to your back. Keep your knees bent all the time. To get back up, bend your knees and roll on to one side. Push up on to your bottom, and swing round on to your hands and knees, from where you can now stand up.

At the end of the book you will find some useful contacts for those with back pain in the UK, as well as a short Recommended Reading list.

CHAPTER 1

Exercise by Prescription

Are you in bed? Right this moment, are you suffering spasms of incapacitating back pain? Wondering how long you'll have to lie there this time? Worrying about when you can get back to work?

We hope not. But if you are, or if the memory of such an incident is still all too fresh in your mind, we believe this book can give you the help you need to end your episodes of back pain once and for all.

Indeed, the long-awaited, highly touted cure for back pain—the treatment that could relieve the agonies of an estimated 80 to 90 percent of the American public and save the country between $16 billion and $50 billion annually in medical expenses and lost work time, according to figures from the American Academy of Orthopædic Surgeons—has actually been discovered. It is called *exercise*. And it works.

Unfortunately, few people really understand the enormous benefits to be gained from exercise, and even fewer people with back pain, therefore, are willing to invest any time or effort in an exercise program specifically aimed at controlling their painful symptoms. Most of the 80 million people who suffer from periodic bouts of back pain continue to think that there must be a more scientific or perhaps even a surgical solution to their woes. They cannot accept the fact that exercise is simply the best, most potent medicine available to treat a back problem.

We consider this lack of knowledge about exercise a national tragedy. The fact is, as little as ten minutes of exercise a day for two weeks will bring about a striking degree of improvement for most people.

When we undertook our landmark study of back pain, we interviewed individuals from all fifty states who had tried literally everything to lead a full life despite a bad back. Our research exploded many popular misconceptions about back care. We showed, for example, that neither orthopedists nor chiropractors usually made the best back doctors, and that the most widely used treatments for back pain were either ineffective or downright dangerous. We also discovered that the right exercises, performed the right way, were the *only* key to a pain-free back.

Our recommendations, published in our book *Backache Relief*, reflected the positive experiences of many survey participants who enjoyed dramatic, long-term relief from back pain, without suffering repeat collapses. What accounted for these individuals' successful outcomes? In a word, *exercise*. The secret to remaining pain-free, they told us, lay in learning —and sticking to—a well-designed exercise program.

The book in your hands outlines just such a safe, sane

exercise program. It gives clear, simple instructions and step-by-step drawings to help you learn the exercise routines with ease. It will also help you devise your own individually tailored exercise program to accomplish any or all of the following goals:

- Prevent back problems from plaguing you in the future
- Treat a disabling episode of acute pain
- Achieve lasting relief from chronic backache
- Make lifestyle changes that can put an end to back pain

Our advice and suggestions about exercise are based not only on our own survey research, but also on our continuing review of recent hospital studies investigating the value of exercise for back pain. Numerous studies, completed since the publication of *Backache Relief*, add further proof that exercise can succeed in helping to alleviate back problems—even after other treatments have failed. Medical researchers all over the world now state confidently that a combination of aerobic, stretching, strengthening, and endurance exercises can bring about genuine improvement for most painful back conditions. Instead of dismissing back pain as "the price we pay for walking upright," specialists are at last coming to see back pain as the consequence of *not walking upright enough*—of spending too much time sitting at the desk, in front of the television, or behind the wheel.

For example, a recent study conducted at the University of Copenhagen, divided 105 patients with chronic low-back pain into three groups. One group underwent three months of intensive exercise training, which entailed thirty workout sessions. The second group attended just as many sessions in the gym, but were asked to perform only a fraction of the activity. The third group had the most sedentary time of all, performing some mild exercise at their sessions, but spending more time receiving heat treatments and massage.

As the doctors reported in 1991 in the journal *Pain*, the subjects in the active-exercise group who continued in training at least once a week over the follow-up year were in the best shape, with less pain and greater mobility than they had at the study's outset. The positive result held as true for women as for men, regardless of age. The researchers also noted that the patient's preexisting conditions had little bearing on their improvement. Indeed, even some veterans of chronic back syndromes got better as a result of the increased activity.

The program we offer in this book is neither rigorous nor difficult. Some of the exercises may seem no more strenuous to you than an everyday activity such as getting out of bed or shopping for your groceries. Yet the simple act of stretching your legs and strengthening your abdominal muscles will have profound effects on the way you look and feel. A small amount of effort will pay off in a noticeable improvement in well-being.

More validation for exercise emerged from a study at Sweden's Sahlgren Hospital. The participants there included 103 industrial workers who had been out of work for eight weeks because of low-back pain. The doctors instructed half of this group in gentle, individually tailored exercises and safety tips for avoiding injury. Not surprisingly, this half wound up going back to work sooner, feeling better. Over the ensuing year, those who exercised and "watched their backs" lost fewer work days than others who did not learn such precautions, according to the researchers' 1992 report in the journal *Physical Therapy*.

In the United States, where back pain accounts for 40 to 50 percent of all lost work days, and as many as one-third of all workers' compensation payments, employees in all sorts of industrial and office settings could be helped by performing exercises at home and learning the back-kindest ways to go about their jobs. You will find tips of this sort in chapters 14, 15, and 16.

When medical studies compare exercise to no exercise, few researchers are surprised to find that the exercise effort paid off in terms of pain relief. Other studies we reviewed went even further in establishing the importance of exercise— by comparing exercise to other widely used treatments for back pain. For example, Dr. Richard A. Deyo of the University of Washington School of Medicine and School of Public Health has tested exercise against transcutaneous electrical nerve stimulation, called TENS. In treatment, the TENS device, about the size of a television remote control, is hooked up to the patient's back via wires and electrodes that gently and steadily jolt the areas of muscle spasm. The electric current is said to confer relaxation and relief. Our own investigation of TENS had convinced us that the units worked —at most—50 percent of the time.

For his research project, Dr. Deyo gave each of his subjects either a real TENS device or a sham TENS unit that gave no jolt but looked like a working machine. Since he never told patients of the differences, each expected some help to come from the little machine. At the same time, Dr. Deyo also put several of the participants on a program of stretching exercise to be performed in addition to the TENS treatments. After one month, the subjects who had exercised were better off than those who hadn't, regardless of whether they had the real or false TENS units. Only the exercise proved valuable. But the subjects didn't seem to understand the connection. Despite the improvement, most of them had quit exercising by the time of the follow-up exam two months later—and their pain had returned.

To help you stick to your exercise program, we've come up with ways to work it into your daily routine, so that you won't look at exercise as just another impossible demand on your time. Chapter 5 gives the details of these strategies, and chapter 6 offers tips on sustaining your motivation to exercise through times when people or problems may tempt you to quit.

Another "treatment" long advocated as a way to beat a bad back is weight control. Doctors have suggested that dieting to lose five to ten pounds would reduce the strain on the back and therefore ward off future episodes of back pain. In our research, we determined that doctors who gave this advice were usually trying to pass the buck—to shift the blame to the patient instead of offering helpful exercise advice. Dr. Deyo later backed us up, when he used national survey data to show that only the very obese stand to gain back-pain relief from losing weight. The person who is just a few pounds above ideal weight is at no greater risk for back trouble than is a thin man or woman. And besides, exercise and increased activity tend to bring weight under reasonable control without the stress of dieting.

Dr. Deyo, who has probably conducted more research into back pain than any other American medical doctor, has also compared exercise to bed rest. He led a series of studies over the last ten years that have helped direct the tide of treatment away from prolonged bed rest and toward an active, healthful lifestyle. He wrote a widely acclaimed report published in 1986 in the *New England Journal of Medicine* that showed two days of bed rest to be sufficient in most cases of back pain. At that time, doctors were routinely recommending two *weeks* in bed for just about any back problem.

Prolonged bed rest for back pain is now recognized as the culprit in causing a host of other unwelcome problems, including bone loss, general weakness, and blood clots in the legs. The risks of prolonged bed rest make it too dangerous a treatment to consider lightly—unless it is attempted as an alternative to an even more dangerous procedure, such as surgery for a ruptured disk.

In other words, even if you are staying home because you have too much pain to go to work, and you cannot manage to sit in a chair, you will probably do better if you spend a good part of each day standing up and resting on your feet, as opposed to staying in bed. In chapter 6 we offer a few preliminary "exercise positions" for people who have been confined to bed by intractable pain, and who are just beginning to be able to exercise.

Further endorsement for exercise activity emerged recently from the so-called Quebec Task Force, a large consortium of researchers and back doctors who reviewed a worldwide collection of clinical reports. They concluded that only two things truly aid the person with common low-back pain: aerobic conditioning (exercise, that is) and education about the proper way to sit, stand, lift, and carry. You will find a guide to appropriate aerobic exercises in chapters 10 and 11, and tips on performing everyday activities, from working at a desk to holding a baby, in chapters 14, 15, and 16.

If you have consulted a doctor about your back pain, you may have received some exercise advice already. We hope so. If, however, your doctor has not mentioned the importance of exercise in alleviating back pain, we urge you to raise the subject yourself. Take this book along to show the doctor, and get his or her opinion of the safety of the program for your specific condition. We feel strongly that the exercises contained here are safe and will pass any practitioner's cautious inspection. We even include, in chapter 11, exercises particularly recommended for specific back-pain conditions, such as osteoarthritis-based back pain and scoliosis. Whatever condition your back is in, you can improve your condition with exercise. Even if you have not been able to exercise in the past, and feel limited by pain now, you can find suggestions in chapter 4 that will help you work a helpful amount of exercise into your life.

CHAPTER 2

Alternatives to Exercise

Exercise is almost invariably better for your back than any-thing else you can put onto or into your body. Compared with all other back-pain treatments, exercise makes the most sense because it is harmless, affordable, and effective.

The same cannot be said of painkillers and anti-inflammatory medications, for example, although these drugs are routinely prescribed for people with back pain. Indeed, drugs constitute the most widely used treatment for back pain. As we discovered in our Back Pain Survey and related research for our book, *Backache Relief,* they do practic-ally no good at all, and their unpleasant side effects may cause considerable harm.

We have said that back pain afflicts an estimated 80 to 90 percent of the population at one time or another, and accounts for somewhere between \$16 billion and \$50 billion annually in medical expenses and lost work time. Many of the treatments that run up these high medical bills are the same ones we are calling ineffective and dangerous. Too many of them have come in and out of fashion like hemlines—proffered at the whim of the practitioners, with no basis in theories of back anatomy and dysfunction. Prolonged bed rest falls into this category. So does traction. So, too, do many varieties of injections and even surgical interventions.

If you are currently suffering from back pain, wondering what course of treatment to pursue or what kind of practitioner to consult, you no doubt have a lot of unanswered questions. Following are the questions we hear most often from people with back problems—along with the answers we've learned from our survey research and our reading of the medical literature.

How long should I rest in bed?
Unless you have a herniated disk, which may require you to stay in bed for a couple of weeks or more, two to four days is now considered ample time to rest a bad back. After that, try to get on your feet and walk around a bit. Sitting may be the last thing you feel like doing.

I want to see a doctor. Could my family doctor help me?
If your family doctor knows you and knows back pain, this may be all the help you'll ever need. If, however, your family doctor's answer to a back problem is to pull out a prescription pad—and this response is all too common among general practitioners—you will no doubt need to look elsewhere. (The pitfalls of prescription pills as a treatment for back pain are discussed in more detail later in this chapter.)

Your family doctor may decide to refer you to a specialist,

such as an orthopedist, a rheumatologist, or a neurosurgeon. Referrals make sense in medicine, so long as the family doctor is really trying to bring in an expert's opinion and assistance—and not merely dismissing you and your back pain by shipping you off to someone else.

General practitioners frequently refer their patients with back pain to an orthopedist, or orthopedic surgeon. Don't let the word *surgeon* scare you. Only about 1 to 3 percent of all cases of back pain can be treated surgically, so the odds of your needing an operation are slim. Instead, a well-informed orthopedist will try to diagnose your condition and prescribe the necessary exercises, or perhaps call in a physical therapist to work with you. An orthopedist who is less well informed—or less inclined to work with people outside the operating room—may say, "There's nothing really wrong with you." This throws the ball back in your court, so to speak, making you feel worse than ever. Now you not only hurt, but you've also been told that you hurt for no good reason. But don't lose hope if this happens to you! This is the time to work out a recovery plan, preferably with your family doctor's help, that involves a graduated program of stretching exercises plus walking.

Do I need X rays to discover what's wrong with my back?
Probably not. The very process of having an X ray may set you up for needless anxiety and disappointment—or worse. Since only a few back conditions show up on X rays, most X-ray findings are negative. In other words, they don't tell you any useful information.

About 80 percent of all cases of low-back pain can be traced to problems with the muscles, ligaments, or disks. And none of these soft tissues show up on an X-ray image. Only bones do.

In some cases, X rays reveal real conditions that may have nothing to do with the current source of pain. Suppose, for example, that you have mild scoliosis, which means that your spine is not perfectly straight. Somehow you have made it through life with no idea of this benign condition. Now that you find yourself in pain, however, some practitioner may be all too ready to blame your discomfort on the scoliosis. It is more likely that you have a muscle spasm or strain, unrelated to the X-ray finding.

Another common X-ray finding in practically anyone over the age of thirty-five is some degree of arthritis in the facet joints of the spine. The odds are still overwhelmingly in favor of your back pain being of a muscular origin—and having an exercise solution.

A real problem with X rays is that doctors who rely on them often conclude, from reading your X ray, that "there's nothing really wrong with you." But really, there *is* something wrong. *It's just that what's wrong with you doesn't show up on the X ray.*

What about chiropractors? Aren't they as good as—or better than—medical doctors for treating back pain?

Chiropractors fared slightly better, at least in the short run, than orthopedists in our Back Pain Survey, which compared and rated more than one hundred types of practitioners and treatments. They enjoyed their greatest success, among our participants, with acute cases of low-back and neck pain. They were less helpful to people who had severe chronic pain; in fact, they often proved counterproductive, as when they attempted to treat conditions such as herniated disk, sciatica, or severe arthritis pain. Likewise, they had little success in correcting scoliosis.

The hands-on manipulation for which chiropractors are famous worked best when it was done gently. Overall, chiropractic manipulation seemed less important, in terms of patient satisfaction, than these practitioners' holistic approach and willingness to listen. Chiropractors dispensed exercise

14

advice as part of their treatments, which was all to the good, and sometimes they gave nutritional counsel as well as advice about lifestyle and the role of stress in aggravating back pain.

Chiropractors, like orthopedists, base their diagnoses on X rays, but, unlike orthopedists, they invariably see a specific cause of pain on an X ray. These causes are termed "subluxa-tions" and "misalignments," often resulting in "pinched nerves," which the chiropractor aims to correct through manipulation of the spine.

The chiropractor's real secret of success, however, is a knowledge of exercise combined with the ability to build a good rapport with patients—and encourage them to exercise.

How can I find out exactly what's wrong with my back?
You may not be able to find out—ever. Our Back Pain Survey showed that practitioners made diagnoses based on their medical specialty and frame of reference. For example, neurol-ogists and rehabilitation doctors frequently recommend an uncomfortable and expensive diagnostic procedure called EMG (electromyography) to check for nerve damage, while orthopedists and primary-care doctors, on the other hand, rarely go this route. This means that two doctors from different fields are more than likely to give you two different names for your condition, and two different explanations of what caused the problem. Or neither one will be able to pinpoint the cause of pain with any specificity.

Although some episodes of back pain can be tied to strains incurred during overexertion or in falls, at least as many bouts strike literally out of the blue. Even if you don't know exactly what laid you up, you can still get better with a brief period of rest followed by devotion to daily exercise.

Who are the back specialists who can help me the most?
The premier back doctor, according to the results of our survey, turned out to be a relatively little-known medical

specialist called a *physiatrist,* or doctor of physical medicine. These practitioners rarely prescribe drugs and do not perform surgery. They prefer instead to use individually prescribed exercise regimens and physical therapy—including ultra-sound (heat) and massage—to treat back pain.

Shouldn't I get some kind of prescription medication?
Probably not. Our survey found no evidence that back sufferers gained any benefit from prescription analgesics (pain pills). Most of these drugs fail to relieve pain; those that do work may be so potent as to upset your stomach and cloud your thinking. If you are taking a drug powerful enough to mute pain, you won't have the warning signal of your pain to guide you, and so you must limit your physical activity in order to avoid further injury. And limiting your activity is ultimately bad for your back.

We found prescription anti-inflammatory drugs to have less value than sugar pills for most cases of back pain—but with far more side effects. Our participants complained of gastrointestinal upsets, including aggravation of ulcers and gastritis. It's not worth taking these drugs, especially when you consider that few back problems even entail inflammation in the first place.

Muscle relaxants, another favorite prescription item, offer some temporary relief to a minority of people with back pain, although these drugs cause potentially dangerous dizziness and drowsiness. Remember that muscles can also be relaxed with physical therapy, heat, massage, and gentle stretching.

Our survey participants found plain old, over-the-counter aspirin to be the most effective drug. And its price was the lowest of all these products.

If you have already received a prescription drug for your back pain, we urge you to discuss this point with your physician.

How do I know if I have a slipped disk? And what treatment will I receive if I do?

Many doctors diagnose a "slipped"—or, more correctly, a "herniated" or ruptured disk—by the degree and location of the patient's pain. This condition frequently causes numbness or tingling in the legs, all the way to the feet. The back, buttock, and leg pain may well be excruciating.

Although herniated disks do not show up on X rays, as explained above, they can be visualized with newer imaging procedures such as CT (computed tomography) scans and MRI (magnetic resonance imaging).

The disks, twenty-two in number, are sandwiched between the upper twenty-four vertebrae of the spinal column, where they cushion the bones and add mechanical strength to the spine. The structure of the disk itself—soft inside, firm outside—invites comparison to a jelly doughnut. An injury or deterioration can make the "jelly" bulge out into the spinal canal, where it may press on a nerve root, causing extreme pain and sometimes threatening paralysis.

A herniated disk is one of the few kinds of backaches that calls for more than two days' bed rest. A herniated disk often—but not always—warrants surgery. Because of the intense pain and the real risk of neurological impairment associated with herniated disk, you will need to seek a medical opinion. Remember, though, that many people have recovered by bed rest alone, or with the aid of strong pain medication. (This is one situation in which such drugs are clearly indicated.)

Since even herniated disks may right themselves, experienced physicians reserve surgery as a last resort, to be avoided until all other, safer approaches—including "tincture of time" in a six-week dose—have failed to deliver relief. Only about 5 to 10 percent of people with herniated disks actually require surgery, according to studies conducted at Harvard Medical School.

Advances in surgical technique have given rise to new, "scarless" disk procedures that can be performed on an outpatient basis, with tiny arthroscopic instruments and lasers. These operations promise fewer complications and faster recuperation at home than result from traditional disk surgery. But the new approaches don't yet match the success rates of the traditional operations. And instead of simply lessening the stress of surgery for those who need it, the seemingly benign procedures are more likely to be offered to people who don't really need surgery.

Manipulation, according to our survey results, is one treatment that can make the pain and disability of a herniated disk considerably worse. Traction is another.

Could my back pain be caused by some other health problem?
It could indeed, and that's why it makes sense to see a medical doctor for a thorough checkup when you have back pain. Conditions that can cause backache include arthritis, kidney disease, colitis, and certain forms of cancer.

I'm a bit overweight. Would dieting help my back pain?
It depends on how overweight you are. Many doctors say that losing five to ten pounds by dieting will reduce the strain on your back and help you avoid future episodes of back pain. But this comment seems to be another "blame the victim" strategy. Studies show that only the very obese stand to gain much pain relief from weight loss. And besides, exercise and increased activity tend to bring weight under reasonable control —*without* dieting.

How can exercise help my back pain?
Exercise stretches and strengthens the four sets of muscles that support the spine. Your abdominal muscles, for example, although they do not attach directly to the spine, are responsi-

ble for girdling your internal organs and contributing to good posture. The abdominals also assist the extensor muscles of the back, which flank the full length of the spine to maintain proper alignment of the vertebrae. Your hip and buttock muscles help support and govern the position of your back while you're sitting, standing, or walking.

Muscle pain typically arises from weakness, spasm or loss of elasticity due to age or inactivity. *All* of these conditions can be remedied through exercise.

A few people I know got over episodes of horrible back pain by trying nutty home remedies, and others got better without doing anything at all about it. So why should I bother exercising?

It's true that many—perhaps most—episodes of intractable back pain end of their own accord, regardless of the treatments applied. The on-again, off-again nature of some back problems, in fact, has given false endorsements to many dubious treatment modalities over the years, from corticosteroid injections to gravity inversion, from TENS to DMSO. Doctors and patients alike may attribute sudden improvement to the treatment of the hour.

Back pain can disappear, in time, with no treatment whatsoever. People who discover this fact for themselves may argue that exercise isn't worth the bother. But exercise can stave off *recurring* bouts of back pain, which tend to grow more debilitating with each successive onset. And back pain that goes away in response to exercise, studies show, tends to return when the exercise is stopped. In other words, your back will thank you for initiating and sticking to a safe exercise program.

19

CHAPTER 3

A Program for Permanent Improvement

By now you understand—intellectually, at any rate—the value of regular exercise in preventing and treating back pain. All that's left is to let us help you devise a personally tailored program that will fit into your life. Adopting the program is a commitment to performing a few stretching and strengthening exercises for ten to fifteen minutes a day—and engaging in aerobic activities for three to four hours a week. This is the biggest lifestyle change the program demands, but, as you'll see, the payoff is measured in an even bigger change in the quality of your life. If you've never exercised regularly before, get ready to feel great!

We urge you to ignore the popular image of exercise as

vigorous and competitive. For back sufferers, as one of our survey participants pointed out, "Slower is generally better, gradual is faster, and vigorous is self-defeating." We might well say, "Any pain, less gain."

All of the back exercises mentioned in this book were performed by the participants in our nationwide Back Pain Survey, who judged them safe and sound. We believe you'll agree. Not every participant performed every exercise, of course—nor should you expect to do so. From the full set, we will help you select those few that best suit your needs, depending on the location, type, severity, and duration of your back pain. Your exercise choices should match your level of fitness, comfort level, time schedule, and tastes. It must enhance your general health, too, so we urge you to check with your doctor about any special restrictions imposed by your personal medical history. Having a wide range of selections from which to choose will not only enable you to personalize your program, but also to change it from time to time—either to make your routine more challenging as you gain experience, or to introduce new exercises just for the sake of variety.

The stretching and strengthening exercises are all explained in detail in chapters 8, 9, and 12, complete with step-by-step instructions and line drawings. The aerobic exercise options are also discussed at length, in chapter 10, with specific suggestions for getting started. Our aim in this chapter is to explain the goals of the different types, and to show how they can work together to promote back fitness.

Your program will consist of three types of exercise:

1. *Aerobic activities*, such as walking and swimming, that increase your stamina and improve your cardiovascular fitness
2. *Stretching exercises*, typified by Knee Drops and Head Rolls, that keep your muscles limber and help prevent spasms

3. *Strengthening exercises,* including Push-offs and Bent-Knee Sit-ups, that firm up the muscles you need to maintain good posture and to carry out everyday activities without putting your back at risk.

Aerobic Exercise

You will spend most of your exercise time engaged in aerobic activities. In fact, aerobic exercise demands a certain minimum time period—at least twenty minutes per session, and preferably forty-five minutes to an hour, repeated three or four times a week. The sustained nature of the activity is what raises your heart rate and gets your blood pumping as you burn oxygen. These effects give aerobic exercise its other well-known name, *cardiovascular activity.* Indeed, the benefits of sustained activity for the heart and circulatory system have by now gained universal acceptance.

But for you, as a person with back trouble, aerobic exercise has another important value: Sustained aerobic activities nourish the disks of your spine by increasing the blood supply to these unique tissues. Much back pain emanates from the disks themselves, which contain abundant nerve endings. To treat your disks well, whether you are trying to protect them from deterioration or help them heal after injury, you do best to pursue aerobic exercise.

The strong relationship between cardiovascular exercise and the health of the spinal disks has implications for other lifestyle choices. You've probably heard at least a million times that smoking is bad for your heart and lungs. But the fact is, smoking damages the disks, too, through its effect on the blood circulation. Nicotine and other components of cigarette smoke compromise the microcirculation—the network of tiny blood vessels throughout the body that feed all the tissues, including the disks. Physicians' surveys have identified cigarette smoking as one of the major risk factors for back pain.

Among backache sufferers, smokers outnumber nonsmokers four to one. And in follow-up studies of people who have undergone operations for the repair of herniated disks, cigarette smokers prove five times more likely to have a poor outcome than postoperative patients who don't smoke.

Alcohol, like cigarette smoke, also constricts the blood vessels and can contribute to poor circulation around the disks. Moderate drinking in social situations probably contributes very little to disk degeneration, but alcohol abuse can aggravate back pain from this source.

You may feel immediate positive effects from aerobic exercise, in addition to backache relief. These could include increased energy during your waking hours, coupled with better sleep at night. You may find that you feel calmer during your aerobic activity period, and that you look forward to this time of day, at least in part, for the stress relief it brings. Over the long term, aerobic exercise will help you shed unwanted pounds, since such activity burns body fat and calories. Provided you don't simultaneously increase your food intake, aerobic exercise will gradually whittle away your excess weight.

Aerobic exercises tend to be everyone's favorites because they are intrinsically enjoyable, or can be made that way. Many of them can be done in the company of others, and therefore provide opportunities for pleasant social contacts. Walking wins our vote for the best aerobic exercise, since it is safe and effective and can be done virtually anytime, anywhere, indoors or out.

Stretching

Your muscles tend to tighten with disuse. If you lead a sedentary life, you can keep your muscles long and limber by intentionally stretching them with exercise. That primes them for action.

24

You probably already know too well what happens when you rely on overly tight muscles to help you make some sudden move: They fail you by going into spasm and slapping you with pain. Now they are in a state of painful contraction, and they may refuse to come out for a long time. The secret of successful treatment for spasm, just like the key to its prevention, lies in gentle stretching.

It's always a good idea to warm up before you stretch. Typical exercise programs for fit people often call for five minutes of jogging in place as a warm-up. But if jogging is too rough for you, or if you are starting out with very limited ability to move, you can warm up in any number of gentler ways. Some of our survey participants reported that they took a warm bath or used a heating pad just before exercise. This enabled them to stretch more readily, get more from the therapy, and increase their rate of progress. If you choose to exercise the very first thing in the morning, you may get an ample warm-up by moving around in bed and then walking for a few minutes before you begin.

When you stretch, try to concentrate on stretching to the point of resistance—and then moving just a fraction beyond it. But, we implore you, *don't push through pain.* Overstretching can be worse than not doing any exercise at all, since it can tear the muscle fibers or induce spasms and pain. Carefully executed back exercises can bring you noticeable improvement in just a few weeks. Please try to be patient. Remember that exercise therapy, no matter how cautious it may seem to you, is almost always better than anything you can put into or onto your body.

Although aerobic exercise can be limited to three or four days a week, stretching does the most for you when you do it every day. This is not just a physiological reality, but a mental one as well; by stretching every day, you make stretching a habit, and you are more likely to stick with it. In chapter 7 we'll discuss other strategies that can help you sustain your motivation to exercise.

25

You may choose to perform all your stretches at once, in a single session, or break up your exercise into two periods, one in the morning and the other at night. The twice-a-day approach works especially well for people who are recovering from an acute episode of back pain, because it helps them make speedier progress. Those who have already attained back fitness, however, and are exercising to maintain the good feeling, can do equally well with a once-a-day regimen.

Each exercise session needs to have its own internal order. After your warm-ups, we suggest you begin with the easiest, gentlest movements, and progress through the more difficult stretching and strengthening exercises. Then cool down by walking at a leisurely pace for about five minutes.

You will notice that many of the stretching and strengthening exercises call for you to make forward-bending movements with your spine, as when you perform the Knee-to-Chest Rock. Exercise experts call this movement *flexion*. Hospital studies have shown that flexion exercises work quickly and effectively to increase the mobility of the lower back.

Another pro-back movement, called *extension*, works to lengthen the spine. You can experience this sensation when you stretch your lower back in executing the Pelvic Tilt.

None of our exercises requires you to hyperextend or arch your back. In both the Cat Stretch and the Head Roll, you have the opportunity to arch your neck, but the instructions tell you to omit this step if neck arching is even the slightest bit uncomfortable. Our exercise philosophy precludes exaggerated arching for two reasons: (1) arching the spine, we believe, puts too much pressure on the disks, and (2) arching the lower back stretches the abdominal muscles.

Regarding the latter, the abdominal muscles really don't require stretching; they have too great a tendency to stretch and sag by themselves. What we really want you to do with your abdominals is build their strength by performing exercis-

26

es such as the Pelvic Tilt, the Bent-Knee Sit-up, and the Sit-Down.

Strengthening

The exercises that build strength in your muscles usually call for you to work against some resistance—to make the muscles work hard so they grow big and strong. It's tempting to think that you can accomplish this goal with aerobic exercise alone, but the fact is you also need specific exercises that call for a short burst of strength from muscle contraction.

Strengthening exercises may be *isotonic* or *isometric*. The isotonic ones involve motion against resistance. For example, in a Push-Off, you push the weight of your body about twelve inches in an effort to strengthen your shoulders and upper back. The isometric exercises involve no obvious movement, just force against resistance. For example, in the Side Press, you push against a wall to strengthen your arm. You may be working just as hard as you did in the Push-Off, but only you can tell how much effort you're expending—since the wall doesn't move.

Fitness enthusiasts who exercise in gyms build strength by lifting weights. We don't include any weight resistance work here, because we feel it's unnecessary for addressing the problem of back pain. Lifting and maneuvering the weight of your own body is sufficient, we feel, for the goals of this program.

Many exercise instructors believe that strengthening exercises should not be done every day. In your back-exercise routine, however, we want you to include them and perform them with the stretches—especially the Pelvic Tilt and Bent-Knee Sit-ups. Unlike weight-resistance exercises, our strengtheners won't tax your body and call for a day or more of rest for muscle repair and recovery between sessions.

27

Instead, these exercises will safeguard your posture and work to reduce your pain.

Sample Exercise Program

The following program is suitable for a person who is reasonably fit, occasionally laid up with back pain, but free of neck pain.

Aerobic activity

Walk for twenty to forty minutes, three times a week.

Stretching

The range of repetitions listed below represents the first day of doing the exercises (the first number) and a month later (the second number).

- Knee-to-Chest (three to six repetitions)
- Knees-to-Chest Rock (two to five repetitions)
- Knee Cross (two to five repetitions each side)
- Cat Stretch (three to six repetitions)
- Knee Spread (two to four repetitions)
- Hamstring Stretch (two to five repetitions each side)
- Thigh Pull (two to four repetitions each side)
- Runner's Stretch (two to four repetitions each side)

Strengthening

The range of repetitions listed below represents the first day of doing the exercises (the first number) and a month later (the second number).

- Pelvic Tilt (five to ten repetitions)
- Bent-Knee Sit-ups (five to ten repetitions)
- Sit-downs (one to five repetitions)

CHAPTER 4

A Special Message for People with Chronically Disabling Back Pain

Our exercise program constitutes a *cure* for 90 percent of people with back pain. But what about the other 10 percent? If you are one of them, please read on.

First, let us assure you that you are not alone. From what we can gather, at least 1.5 million Americans, and perhaps as many as 5 million, are severely disabled by back pain that has resisted every treatment brought to bear. Some of these individuals have what physicians call "Failed Back Syndrome." This is an unfortunate euphemism for a poor surgical outcome from diskectomy or other operation on the spine. The term makes it sound as though the patient's back were guilty of some kind of gross failure, when really it is the surgery or other treatments that failed to bring improvement to the person. The individual continues to suffer, but with less hope than before, and the hope diminishes as the realization grows that no help may be forthcoming from any source.

Even without surgery, some backache sufferers find themselves growing progressively worse, no matter what they do. We want to tell you about one of these people, a participant in our original Back Pain Survey, who suffered the kind of anguish you may be going through.

When he filled out his survey questionnaire, Bob had seen both orthopedists and chiropractors, as well as osteopaths, naturopaths, and numerous other conventional and alternative health practitioners. No two of his twelve diagnoses were the same, so he never knew what was wrong with his back. Still, he continued to read widely about back pain, to seek professional help, and try each new seemingly sound and rational remedy.

In a page he stapled onto the survey, Bob described his predicament:

> Some doctors who know about the chronicity of my problem won't even allow me to make an appointment to see them. If they do agree to examine me, they're all but itching to get me out the door. It is assumed that I have workmen's compensation or some other kind of insurance, which I don't, or that I'm a neurotic who enjoys the attention. Actually, I live alone, and nobody pays me any attention unless I'm up and about. Some people obviously think I'm a malingerer, even though I worked from age fourteen to forty. It's just been the past five years that I've not been able to be on my feet long enough to hold down a job. I am living off my savings, which are about depleted.

The questionnaire explained that the information people provided would be used in a book we were writing about back pain (*Backache Relief*, Times Books 1985, NAL/Signet 1986).

Bob was a little concerned about that. In a postscript he added, "I hope that your book won't leave out people like me. I hope it won't be another simplistic *Six Minutes a Day to Relief*, full of 'guaranteed safe' exercises I can't even do."

We did not leave Bob out of our first book, and we won't leave him—or you—out of this one, either.

If you are suffering from long-standing, seemingly intractable back problems, you may require special preparations or expert exercise guidance from a trained practitioner before you can make use of the exercises we describe in subsequent chapters. Bob, when we last heard from him, had started to find his way out of that prolonged disability, and to look forward to functioning normally once again.

What follows are some suggestions on fighting your way back from extreme disability over a long period of time.

Try seeing a physiatrist.
Even if you have a long list of professionals you've already consulted, you may do well to take your troubles to a doctor of physical medicine and rehabilitation, also known as a physiatrist. These practitioners are accustomed to treating debilitating conditions, from spinal cord injuries to strokes, and are not easily frightened off by pain that has a long history. They are not trained as surgeons, although they can spot problems that do require surgical treatment, and then make appropriate referrals. Physiatrists recognize the value of exercise, and have a thorough knowledge of exercise as a prescription drug. Of all the medical specialists, the physiatrist is the most likely to be able to create an individualized exercise program that promises gradual improvement.

Another thing a physiatrist will likely do for you is to recommend physical therapy. The physical therapist, acting under the doctor's orders, will work with you on the successful execution of your exercises, as well as give you treatments that could include heat, or massage, or both.

In the UK, we do not have an equivalent of the US physiatrist. Instead, the closest practitioner is likely to be a doctor who specializes in rehabilitating those who have suffered from debilitating pain and disease, including those with chronic back pain. You can talk to your GP about whether or not you could be referred for such specialist treatment. If your condition is suitable, your GP will also refer you for physiotherapy.

Make a plan for achieving progress slowly.
If your back pain has been growing worse over a period of years, you can't really expect to finally hit on one solution that will solve your problems and land you back on your feet overnight. Anyone who promises you that kind of outcome has to be lying.

Accept the fact that your recovery may take as long as a year, and promise yourself that by the end of the year you will have made substantial progress. And then set out to make that promise come true the way several of our survey participants did—gradually. *Very* gradually.

Perhaps you can be out of bed only a few minutes a day. Try to stop blaming yourself for being incapacitated. Instead of fixating on all the things you used to do that you can't do now, look on those daily minutes out of bed as an indication that you have made some progress and can make much more. Time yourself when you're out of bed so that you know exactly what you can do—the precise number of minutes and seconds that you are up and about. Tell yourself, "Tomorrow I can manage one minute more than that." Just one more minute. One more minute of standing or walking. When you reach that goal, enjoy your success, rather than belittling your achievement as small or insignificant. In just one month, one minute a day translates into half an hour more per day—and thirty more successes. In two months you've gained an hour, and by year's end, six hours. Long before the year is out, you'll be ready for the pre-exercise positions in chapter 6, and then for a simple program of gentle movements to start a lifelong program of regular exercise.

Try to reduce the stress of incapacitation.
Being out of work, out of the swim, breeds its own stress. Being in pain is stressful. But stress, in turn, can often aggravate pain, setting up a vicious circle of emotional and physical anguish. If you have neck pain, you may be especially vulnerable to aggravation of pain by stress. Knowing the role stress can play for someone with long-standing backache, please consider the stress-reduction strategies in chapter 13 as being of particular importance for you.

Make your environment work for you.
You may feel "trapped" by your disability, and rail against the four walls. But there may be many small changes you can make in your surroundings that will collectively contribute to an improvement in your condition. To take the most obvious example, namely the bed you're lying in, ask yourself if the mattress is really firm and comfortable. Are you supporting your body with pillows to your best advantage? If you're watching television, is the set positioned so that you can see the screen without straining your neck or body alignment? Even if you're not carrying out your normal daily activities now, check the suggestions in chapters 14, 15, and 16 to discover ideas about back-safe strategies for doing a variety of everyday tasks. If you follow these suggestions as you make progress, you can avoid further injury.

Remember that your attitude about your body is the basis for improvement.
By celebrating each small success and making your environment as pleasant as possible, you are respecting and nurturing your body. In time, your pain will lessen and you will be able

to do many more things. Believe it or not, you have an advantage over many other backache sufferers, and that is that you will never take your recovery for granted. Once you regain your ability to move, you will take such joy in movement that no one will ever have to nag you to exercise. No doubt you will look forward to that fifteen or twenty minutes a day spent exercising as quality time when you are alone, quiet, in touch with yourself, meditative, knowing that you are doing something good for yourself. And because you have that attitude, you can look forward to keeping yourself well.

P A R T
T W O

The Motivation

> *Once people accept exercise as medicine, the hardest thing is to get them to take that medicine regularly.*

CHAPTER 5

How to Work Exercise into Your Life

Exercise is a life-transforming tool for back sufferers that will make more of a difference in your sense of well-being than anything else—including the best food, the greatest sex, the most exhilarating fun. The only catch is that you have to do it to reap the benefits.

If you're like most busy people, you already have too much to do. There isn't room in your day for even fifteen minutes of stretching and strengthening exercises, let alone the forty-five minutes to an hour, three times a week, that would satisfy the aerobic exercise requirement of our program.

We're going to help you find the time—somehow—because, again, we are confident that exercise will prove more beneficial to you in the long run than any other approach you can try.

Let's start with the argument that you just don't have any time. Well, then, you certainly don't have time to spend three days in bed, do you? What if we told you that the relatively small time commitment to exercise could buy you an insurance policy against the next time you might have to call in sick to work because "My back has gone out again"?

If time is money, then the time you invest in exercise, which costs you nothing, saves you whatever amount of money you could conceivably spend on chiropractic adjustments, X rays, or prescription medications your family doctor prescribes—the next time your back muscles seize up and lay you low.

What's that? You say you're already running so flat-out that you can't give yourself enough sleep at night, and so you're tired all day? That's no excuse, either. As you'll see, exercise, especially regular aerobic exercise, will change the way you feel, every minute of the day. Instead of depleting your energy, as you might suppose, exercise actually gives you more energy. Even though it burns up calories and cuts through fat on your body, it doesn't make you tired. On the contrary, exercise makes you feel more alert and alive—and because you tend to sleep better when you exercise, you're likely to find that you feel more rested even when you spend fewer hours in bed.

Maybe these arguments sound too pat. We set up a straw man, then knock it down, but meanwhile, you really are too busy to exercise. Let's try another approach. Let's look at your day and see if there's someplace, any place, that we can squeeze in the requisite amount of exercise. Maybe you can do your exercises while you're watching your children or warming food in the microwave. If you can allow for three five-minute mini-exercise sessions spread over the course of the day, you'll benefit from even that much, we promise. So ask yourself the following questions, and maybe you'll find the answer to the problem of not having time to exercise.

If you work at a regular job . . .
Can you walk to work instead of driving or taking public transportation?

Do you have time to walk on your lunch hour?

Is there a health club or a pool near your workplace where you can swim during your lunch hour?

If you work in a building that has several floors, can you climb the steps instead of riding the elevator?

Can you interest your employer in starting a "back school" to help your co-workers learn exercise and back-friendly work habits on the job?

Honestly, if while sitting at your desk, you went through the whole series of neck-stretching exercises, from Left-Right to Head Pull, would anyone think you were doing anything so terribly strange?

Couldn't you also get away with performing most of the neck-strengthening exercises, as well as the routine for the shoulders and upper back?

If you need to talk to a colleague in the building, would you consider walking there for a face-to-face conference instead of dialing his or her extension on the telephone?

If you work at home . . .
Isn't it possible to lie down on the floor and stretch your back while you're taking a respite shorter than a coffee break?

Since no one's around to watch you, can you do your neck exercises while you're on the telephone? (That way, you'll avoid doing something to hurt your neck, such as cradling the phone between your ear and your shoulder for too many minutes at a time.)

When it's time to check the mailbox or go to the post office, can you walk for twenty minutes?

If you are caring for young children . . .
Wouldn't the baby love to go for a long walk in the stroller?

Can the baby play or nap on a quilt on the floor while you do your routine lying down nearby?

Why not make your exercises a family activity? Or a game like "Simon Says"?

Can you walk briskly along with your older children while they ride their bikes?

If you are doing housework . . .
Can you find opportunities to make every chore a stretch? (This may involve putting aside some of your labor-saving devices in favor of doing things the old-fashioned way, such as hanging laundry on a line.)

If your house has more than one level, would you mind making several trips up and down for the laundry? (Taking the steps more frequently would probably be better for your back than struggling to carry a heavy load either up or down.)

If you own your own home . . .
Can you turn fall leaf-raking, winter snow-shoveling, and summer lawn care and gardening into aerobic activities? (If so, be sure to approach these activities safely, following the tips in chapter 15.)

If you enjoy soaking in the tub every evening . . .
Can you execute a Pelvic Tilt underwater?

How about a Bent-Knee Sit-up?

Would you believe that exercising in a warm tub can be especially soothing?

If all else fails . . .
Would you consider carrying out your neck, upper back, and standing back exercises in the shower?

Can you find five minutes, three times a day, to lie down on the floor and stretch your muscles? (Watch for opportunities, such as when you're waiting for some family member to get out of the bathroom, or for the stove timer to tell you that dinner is ready, or for your favorite television program to begin.)

Can you find a friend who also needs to exercise, and who'll visit with you while you both walk aerobically?

With the above possibilities in mind, can you create your own opportunities to give yourself the benefit of regular exercise? You can. Of course you can.

CHAPTER 6

How to Assess Your Exercise Readiness and Assemble Your Tailor-Made Program

Now that you're motivated to exercise—aware of all the pain-relieving, mobility-increasing benefits a program of regular exercise can bring you—you're ready to begin selecting the elements of your individually tailored exercise routine.

In this chapter, we want to help you determine your level of exercise ability, based on factors such as your age, your assessment of your own general fitness, and the duration of your back pain. Then we can make specific exercise suggestions. An "off-the-rack" exercise program cannot possibly suit you as well as a program designed with your needs in mind.

The nature of your back problem also guides you in identifying the ideal exercises for you. As we've said earlier, few people can give a specific name or diagnosis to their back pain. Nevertheless, certain identifiable conditions, including sciatica and osteoarthritis-induced back pain, call for particular precautions.

Let's begin with a simple self-test that will match your level of back pain and limitation with a reasonable set of exercise goals.

SELF-TEST OF EXERCISE READINESS

Please circle the number that best completes each of the following statements:

Most days, I am . . .
- (1) inactive because of pain or chronic disability
- (2) inactive by choice—a "couch potato"
- (3) moderately active
- (4) very active

When I get up in the morning, I feel . . .
- (1) severe pain that never seems to go away completely
- (2) pain that warns me to be careful
- (3) pain on some days, no pain on others
- (4) hardly any pain at all

As I go through the day, I find that I . . .
- (1) need most things done for me
- (2) need help to do some things
- (3) manage well on my own, if I'm careful of my back
- (4) can keep up a normal pace of activity, at work and/or at home, with comfort

My back pain stems from . . .
   (1) osteoarthritis, or herniated disk, or sciatica
   (2) an accident that injured my back some time ago
   (3) muscle spasms
   (4) some unknown cause

Because of my back pain . . .
   (1) I've had surgery at least once
   (2) I've been confined to bed several times, and am some-
       what limited in the things I can do
   (3) I've had to stay in bed on occasion, but between
       episodes of pain I get along fine
   (4) I may think twice before I try some new activity, but I
       can pretty much do what I want

**My experience with exercise in general and back exercise
in particular is . . .**
   (1) nonexistent
   (2) limited
   (3) moderate
   (4) extensive

My age is . . .
   (1) over sixty-five
   (2) mid-fifties to early sixties
   (3) early forties to mid-fifties
   (4) forty or younger

   Now we'd like you to classify yourself in one of four
categories, based on your responses to the above questionnaire items. If you circled all ones, for example, or mostly

ones, then you are in the "Basic Preparation" category. If your answers included more twos than ones, consider yourself in the "Proceed With Caution" group. If you found the threes to be most descriptive of your condition, please put yourself in the "Gentle Exercise" category. If you scored fours consistently, you are no doubt ready for the "Regular Exercise" category.

Over time, as you make progress and change your level of flexibility and strength, you may move on through the categories at whatever pace seems right for you. There is nothing to stop a person who begins in the Basic Preparation Category from becoming a Regular Exerciser. Indeed, by preparing for exercise and then proceeding with caution at first, you can *expect* to progress to Gentle Exercise and finally to Regular Exercise. And you needn't stop there.

Basic Preparation
(Category 1)

If you suffer from a case of chronically debilitating back pain, please see the special message in chapter 4 before you read on. We have every confidence that you will be able to use the exercises in this book, but first we want to prepare you to perform them safely.

If you are just now recuperating from an acute episode of debilitating back pain, you can try the following pre-exercise positions as soon as your contracted muscles have eased enough for you to move around in bed—or be up and about for just a few minutes at a time. These are such conservative movements that they are safe to attempt *before* your pain lessens enough to permit other exercises. Give yourself a week or two of assuming these positions, in bed, as meaningful first steps toward full activity.

Start slowly and hopefully. There's no need to do all of the positions in one session, or even all in one day at the outset. If you can be comfortable in the Basic Exercise Position for five minutes the first time you try it, move on to the Pelvic Lift later in the day or the next morning. Once you master the Pelvic Lift, and can assume that position for ten minutes at a time, twice a day, you may attempt the Knee Clasp.

BASIC EXERCISE POSITION

If you have been in severe pain, the muscles and ligaments in your lower back have no doubt contracted, creating an exaggerated "S" curve there. Holding the Basic Exercise Position for several minutes will begin to correct that painful swayback, or lordosis. You can gauge the amount of correction each time you slip your hand under the small of your back.

Starting position: Assume the fetal position, lying on your side with both knees bent. *a*

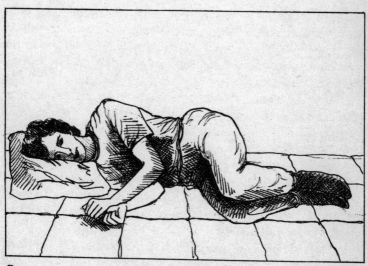

a

Steps:
1. Roll onto your back, and place your arms at your sides. *b*
2. Position your feet flat on the mattress, with your heels about six to eighteen inches from your buttocks.
3. Hold this position for about two minutes.
4. Slip one hand, palm down, between the small of your back and your mattress. *c*
5. Remove your hand, and lie in the Basic Exercise Position another two or three more minutes.
6. Repeat Step 4. You'll likely find there's a bit less room for your hand, now that you've been lying flat a longer time.
7. Return to the starting position.

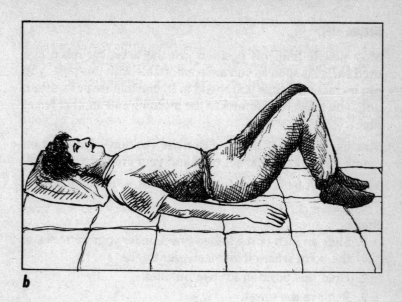

b

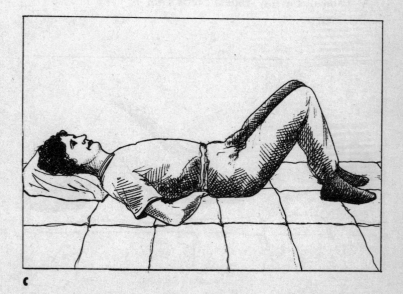

c

PELVIC LIFT

Most people find this position just the ticket for relaxing a tired back. As soon as you are comfortable with this pose, you can increase the time you spend in it, one minute per session, until you reach ten minutes in the morning and another ten at night.

Starting position: The Basic Exercise Position—lying flat on your back with your knees bent and your arms at your sides.

Materials: A bath towel, folded just once, so that it is not too bulky.

Steps:
1. Slide an inch of the folded towel under your buttocks, at the point where they meet your thighs.
2. Hold this position for two minutes.
3. Remove the towel.
4. Later in the day, repeat Steps 1–3.

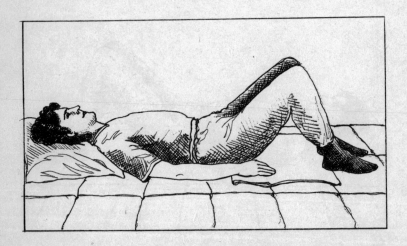

KNEE CLASP

These maneuvers are starting to feel like bona fide exercises. Please remember that the point of this stretch is to let you relax in a comfortably flexed position—and not to challenge you to draw your knees toward your chest as far as you possibly can.

Starting position: The Pelvic Lift Position—lying flat on your back with knees bent, arms at your sides, and a folded towel just under your buttocks. *a*

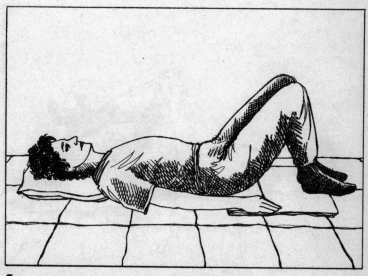

a

Steps:

1. Bring one knee up toward your chest and hold it there with your hand. **b**
2. Bring the other knee up. **c**
3. Clasp your hands together, holding your knees just below the kneecaps.
4. As gently as you can, pull your knees a few inches toward your chest. **d**
5. Hold this position for a count of six.
6. Return to the starting position.
7. Repeat Steps 1–6 six times.

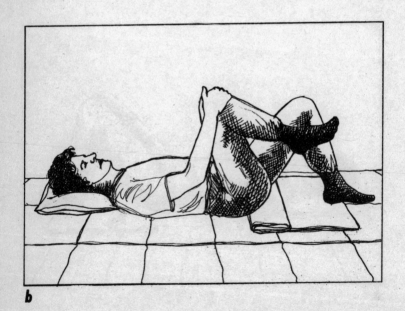

b

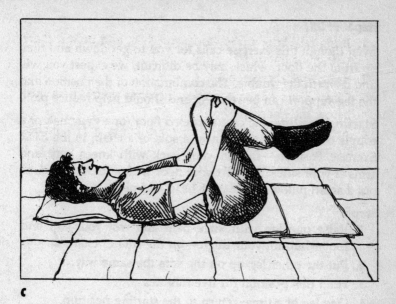

c

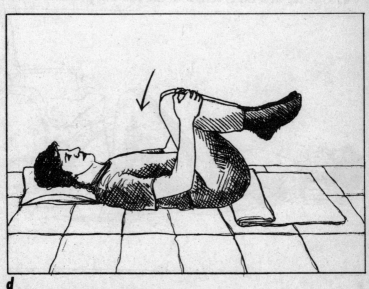

d

LEG SUPPORT

Even though this exercise calls for you to get down and then up from the floor, which may be difficult, we expect you will find it worth the trouble. The combination of the position and the leg support can be relaxing and should help reduce pain.

Starting position: Lie on a carpeted floor (or a gym mat, or a couple of folded blankets) near a sofa or a chair, in the Basic Exercise Position—flat on your back with knees bent and arms at your sides. Support your neck with a folded towel, or put a small pillow under your head and neck. *a*

Steps:
1. Raise one leg with knee bent and rest your calf and foot—but not your thigh—on the sofa or chair. *b*
2. Put the other leg up on the sofa the same way. *c*
3. Hold this position for five minutes.
4. One leg at a time, return to the starting position.

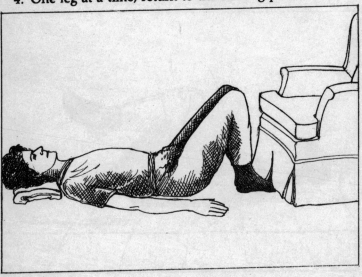

a

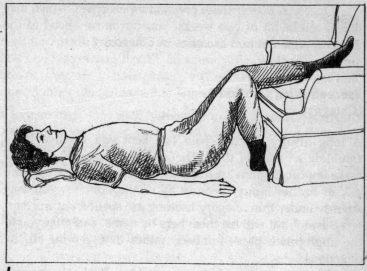

b

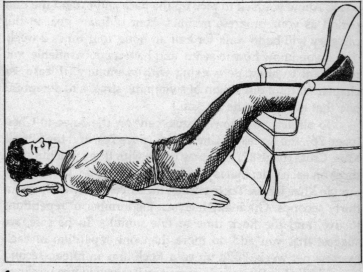

c

Once you master these preparatory exercises, which may take a minimum of two weeks, you can move ahead to the Proceed With Caution exercises in Category 2.

Proceed With Caution (Category 2)

A long history of back pain has kept you inactive for a troubling amount of time. The exercises that will help you make important gains are necessarily gentle ones that carry no risk of further injury. Because all of the exercises you may attempt under this category heading are spelled out in chapters 8 and 9, we will list them here by name, and refer you to the appropriate page numbers, rather than reprint all the directions.

For your aerobic activity, try walking. Begin slowly, and for a maximum of twenty minutes at a time, three times a week. Allow yourself to pick up the pace and extend the time period as your progress permits. Your ultimate goal in this category will be to walk for half an hour, four times a week.

If you know how to swim, and have a pool available, you may want to alternate walking with swimming. (Please see chapter 10 for a discussion of swimming strokes to determine one that is appropriate for you.)

To stretch your lower back, rely on the Knee-to-Chest (page 76), the Knees-to-Chest Rock (page 74), and the Simple Knee Cross (page 82). You may begin with three repetitions— three on each side, that is—of both the Knee-to-Chest and the Simple Knee Cross. Try to sustain the Knees-to-Chest Rock for thirty seconds. Gradually increase the number of repetitions to five, and the Rock time to one minute. To be safe, we suggest that you add no more than one repetition of each exercise per week. Build up your Rock time in fifteen-second increments. In other words, it may well take you two weeks or longer to go from three to five repetitions, from thirty seconds to one minute.

To strengthen your abdominal muscles, practice five repetitions of the Pelvic Tilt (page 91). As you gain strength, you may build up to ten repetitions. The same holds true for the Standing Pelvic Tilt (page 93). Also attempt the Bent-Knee Sit-ups (page 96), starting with three repetitions a day, and gradually building to ten.

For your buttocks, hips, and legs, rely on The Squeeze (page 98), the Knee Spread (page 98), and the Hip Hikers (page 103), starting with three repetitions of each one every day and building gradually to five.

If you need to stretch the muscles of your neck, try doing the Left-Right (page 113), the Yes-No (page 114), and the Neck Tilt (page 120). It's safe to begin with three repetitions of each, then build to five. To strengthen the muscles of your neck, we recommend the Bed Head (page 121), beginning with three repetitions and moving up to five.

Stretch your shoulders and upper back with the Prone Shoulder Stretch (page 124) and the Shoulder Shrug (page 125). Start at three repetitions and progress to five at the usual pace. Strengthen the upper back area with the Side Press (page 133).

As you gain flexibility in this stage of your program, keep reminding yourself of the good progress you're making. It has taken you a long time to lose and then regain your sense of well-being, so we urge you to let yourself enjoy every aspect of improvement.

After several weeks of slow and steady progress have brought you to the completion of the Category 2 goals, you need not rush ahead to the next level. By all means, let your own assessment of your condition be your guide. You may want to approach Category 3 by taking just a few new exercises and incorporating them into the routine you're following now. On the other hand, you may switch to the

Category 3 exercises, holding on to those elements of Category 2 that seem particularly helpful to you.

Proceed With Caution

Knee-to-Chest (page 76)
Total Body Relaxation (page 158)
Knees-to-Chest Rock (page 74)
Simple Knee Cross (page 82)
Pelvic Tilt (page 91)
Standing Pelvic Tilt (page 93)
Bent-Knee Sit-ups (page 96)
The Squeeze (page 98)
Knee Spread (page 98)
Hip Hikers (page 103)
Left-Right (page 113)
Yes-No (page 114)
Neck Tilt (page 120)
Bed Head (page 121)
Prone Shoulder Stretch (page 124)
Shoulder Shrug (page 125)
Side Press (page 133)

Gentle Exercise
(Category 3)

Because you are already fairly active and relatively pain-free, you can attempt a variety of movements. We encourage you to walk for fitness, or alternate swimming with walking, so that you give yourself a forty-minute aerobic workout at least four times a week. If time allows, and as your sense of yourself dictates, you can work up to six sessions per week of aerobic activity, each session lasting as long as an hour. We'd like you to set the pace of this activity at a comfortable level. In other words, when you walk, walk with purpose and direction as though you have somewhere to go—but *not* as though you have to rush because you're late for an appointment.

Work on stretching your lower back with five repetitions of the following six exercises: Knee-to-Chest (page 76), Double Knee-to-Chest (page 78), Knee Drops (page 79), Knee Cross (page 84), Flexibility Twist (page 162) and Twists and Tilts (page 89). If you are comfortable with these movements, you may increase the number of repetitions, one at a time, every three or four days, until you reach ten.

Strengthen your abdominal muscles with five repetitions each of the Pelvic Tilt (page 91), the Standing Pelvic Tilt (page 93), and the Bent-Knee Sit-ups (page 96). At the same pace as you increase your repetitions of stretching exercises, add repetitions of these movements, too, up to ten.

Work your buttocks, hips, and legs by attempting five repetitions of these four exercises: Knee Spread (page 98), Hamstring Stretch (page 100), Thigh Pull (page 104), and Runner's Stretch (page 108). Here, too, slowly work your way up to ten repetitions.

If you have tight neck muscles, loosen them with five daily repetitions of these three exercises: Left-Right Plus (page 114), Neck Bob (page 116), and Head Pull (page 119). Progressing gradually along with the rest of the regimen, you can increase the number of repetitions to ten.

Try to strengthen your neck with three repetitions each of the Neck Push (page 122) and Side Neck Push (page 123). Work up to five repetitions of each.

For stretching your shoulders and upper back, rely on the Shoulder Shrug (page 125), Shoulder Roll (page 126), and Airplane (page 130). Try beginning with three repetitions of each, then working up to five. For stretching these same areas, begin with three repetitions each of the Push-offs (page 132) and the Side Press (page 133), then gradually work toward five repetitions.

By the time you arrive at the full recommended number of repetitions in this category, you will be enjoying a greater range of motion, and probably less anxiety about suffering a relapse of back pain. At this point, you're ready for "Regular Exercise," which has a little more oomph.

Gentle Exercise

> Total Body Relaxation (page 158)
> Knee-to-Chest (page 76)
> Double Knee-to-Chest (page 78)
> Knee Drops (page 79)
> Knee Cross (page 84)
> Flexibility Twist (page 162)
> Twists and Tilts (page 89)
> Pelvic Tilt (page 91)
> Standing Pelvic Tilt (page 93)
> Bent-Knee Sit-ups (page 96)
> Knee Spread (page 98)
> Hamstring Stretch (page 100)
> Thigh Pull (page 104)
> Runner's Stretch (page 108)
> Left-Right Plus (page 114)
> Neck Bob (page 116)
> Head Pull (page 119)
> Neck Push (page 122)
> Side Neck Push (page 123)
> Shoulder Shrug (page 125)
> Shoulder Roll (page 126)
> Airplane (page 130)
> Push-offs (page 132)
> Side Press (page 133)

Regular Exercise
(Category 4)

Since you are on your feet and free of pain most of the time, you probably perform exercises as insurance against future episodes of back pain. Good for you! Indeed, from your active vantage point, some of these exercises may look too simple. But please don't scoff at them. They serve the important function of focusing on the very muscles and movements that ward off back troubles. Remember, you never outgrow your need for the Pelvic Tilt!

If you crave action, start pulling out the stops in your aerobic exercise. When you walk, go quickly. Swing your arms. You can even pump them to push up your heart rate and pep up your pace. Swim if you like. And try an exercise bike or ride a bike outdoors for an aerobic alternative.

In stretching your lower back, you may use any or all of the exercises in chapter 8. Begin with five repetitions of six of them: Knee-to-Chest (page 76), Knees-to-Chest Rock (page 74), Knee Cross (page 84), Cat Stretch (page 86), Flexibility Twist (page 162), and Twists and Tilts (page 89). Increase the number of repetitions every three or four days, until you are doing ten of each.

For abdominal strengthening, go for the Pelvic Tilt (page 91), Standing Pelvic Tilt (page 93), Bent-Knee Sit-ups (page 96), and Sit-downs (page 94). Here, too, start with five repetitions of each and work up to ten.

Stretch and strengthen your buttocks, hips, and legs with the Knee Spread (page 98), Hamstring Stretch (page 100), Hip Hikers (page 103), Standing Thigh Pull (page 106) and Runner's Stretch (page 108). Try five repetitions of each for starters, then work up to ten.

Neck-stretching exercises for you could include five repetitions each of Left-Right Plus (page 114), Neck Bob (page 116), Head Roll (page 117), and Head Pull (page 119). Work up to ten of each of these over time.

Strengthen your neck with the Bed Head (page 121), Neck Push (page 122), and Side Neck Push (page 123), beginning with three and working up to five repetitions of each.

To stretch your shoulders and upper back, start out with three repetitions each of the Shoulder Roll (page 126), Roller

Blades (page 128), Square Shoulder Stretch (page 129), Airplane (page 130), and Windmill (page 131). As you gain proficiency with these, increase the number of repetitions to five. Strengthen these areas with five Push-offs (page 132) and three Side Presses (page 133), gradually increasing to ten repetitions and five repetitions respectively. For your hamstrings, try the Sitting Spine Stretch (page 159).

Regular Exercise

Total Body Relaxation (page 158)
Knee-to-Chest (page 76)
Knees-to-Chest Rock (page 74)
Knee Cross (page 84)
Cat Stretch (page 86)
Flexibility Twist (page 162)
Twists and Tilts (page 89)
Pelvic Tilt (page 91)
Standing Pelvic Tilt (page 93)
Bent-Knee Sit-ups (page 96)
Sit-downs (page 94)
Knee Spread (page 98)
Hamstring Stretch (page 100)
Hip Hikers (page 103)
Standing Thigh Pull (page 106)
Runner's Stretch (page 108)
Left-Right Plus (page 114)
Neck Bob (page 116)
Head Roll (page 117)
Head Pull (page 119)
Bed Head (page 121)
Neck Push (page 122)
Side Neck Push (page 123)
Shoulder Roll (page 126)
Roller Blades (page 128)

Square Shoulder Stretch (page 129)
Airplane (page 130)
Windmill (page 131)
Push-offs (page 132)
Side Press (page 133)
Sitting Spine Stretch (page 159)

That's all you have to do, really, to safeguard your back through exercise. Except that you need to keep doing your exercises. And please don't forget to go about your normal activities in a back-friendly frame of mind—even when your back forgets to remind you. You're getting to the point at which you can tell people that your back *used to be* a problem.

You can use the following form to record your own exercise plan, and then keep track of additions and changes. This is a good way to mark your progress and to troubleshoot for the causes of later soreness, but if it seems like too much paperwork for you, by all means just move on to the next chapter.

BACK EXERCISE PROGRESS CHART

Week #   Day #

Aerobic activity _____   Length of time _____

Stretching and Strengthening Exercises

Exercise	Repetitions	Notes
_____	_____	_____
_____	_____	_____
_____	_____	_____
_____	_____	_____
_____	_____	_____
_____	_____	_____
_____	_____	_____
_____	_____	_____
_____	_____	_____
_____	_____	_____
_____	_____	_____
_____	_____	_____
_____	_____	_____
_____	_____	_____
_____	_____	_____

CHAPTER 7

How to Sustain Your Motivation to Exercise

You are your own best judge of the strategies that will work to keep your motivation and your body primed to exercise. After all, who knows you better? Are you the persevering sort who feels duty-bound to stick with every new resolution? Or are you in danger of losing interest in this exercise endeavor during the several weeks it may take for you to see gratifying results? Are you a loner who will eagerly set out for an early-morning walk before going to work? Or do you prefer a social setting in which to exercise—walking with a group of friends, perhaps, or working out at a gym?

Pain and disability may be the chief motivating factors right now, but your attention to exercise is likely to relieve pain and help you become active again. Then what? Numerous studies in hospitals have shown that even when people get back on their feet because of exercise, they tend to drop the program within a few months, perhaps out of a sense of false security. They don't think they could wind up in bed in pain again. But, unfortunately, statistics prove them wrong. Dropping the exercise that made them well turns out to be an invitation for pain and spasm to return. And it often returns with a vengeance.

If our program of exercise is to be of any lasting benefit, we have to give you ways to sustain it indefinitely. We have to persuade you to stick with your exercise regimen through good times and bad—through family crises, during illness, on vacations, while traveling for business, and regardless of any other situation that tempts you to forget about exercise for a while.

How to Reinforce Your Plan to Exercise Every Day

• Keep a log of your exercise progress—*and* the improvements in your condition, including increased mobility and decreased pain. That way, you'll have a written reminder of the reasons to stay with the program.

• Set aside a place for performing your exercise routine. Keep everything you need handy—a towel, a mat, a special warm-up suit, or whatever else you've decided you need. Then you can get right to work during your allotted time. If you live in cramped quarters and can't create a designated exercise area, then put all the items into a shopping bag and stow it close to your favorite workout spot.

• Schedule a time of day that you regularly devote to exercise. Treat that time like a business meeting or a family outing. In other words, it's important time, and other things can't be allowed to interfere with it. (On those rare occasions when you can't stick to your set time, it's much better to find another time rather than lose that day of exercise. But if you have to miss a day because of illness, it won't set back your progress.)

• Sit down and write yourself a letter in which you explain all your exercise goals and hopes for improvement. Put the letter away in a safe place. You may never need to look at it again, but if you find yourself looking for excuses to avoid exercise, take out the letter and read it.

How to Keep Your Exercise Period Free of Distractions

• Choose a time of day when you're least likely to be disturbed.

• Ignore the telephone if it rings.

• Put a note on your door telling people that you will be right back, and that they should not bother ringing the bell.

• Play some pleasing music that will cover any extraneous, distracting sounds. The music may also help you keep count where you need to count, and move gracefully in time to the music.

How to Get Others to Help You Stick to Your Program

• Arrange to exercise regularly with a friend or two. This puts your exercise in a social context, which may make the activity more pleasant for you. What's more, when you're tempted to skip a day, you won't want to back out and disappoint your friends, will you?

• Ask your doctor to compile a list of your vital statistics. This should include your weight, pulse, blood pressure, and cholesterol level, including the percentage of high- and low-density lipoproteins. Ask your doctor to recheck the measurements periodically, say every three or four months. You'll see documented evidence that you're shedding extra pounds, that your resting pulse may be slowing down the way an athlete's does, that your blood pressure is within normal limits, and that your cholesterol level stays in the low range.

• Enlist your children's cooperation, if they are old enough to understand, by explaining that your exercise time is important to your health, and that you want them to keep themselves occupied while you work out. If they're too young for such tactics, you can try to schedule your exercise period during the times when your infant naps or after your toddler has gone to bed. Another possibility is to let your youngsters join your activity: While you stretch and strengthen, they can work their bodies, too—practicing somersaults or other gymnastics.

How to Take Your Exercise Program on the Road

• When you plan to visit an out-of-town hotel, whether for vacation or a business trip, inquire about exercise facilities. Many hotels and motels now have equipment rooms with treadmills for walking and exercise bikes for riding. The swimming pool, assuming there is one, may give you an opportunity you don't usually have to work in some swimming. Some hotels offer walking/jogging maps of the neighborhood.

• Since your back-stretching and strengthening exercises require no special equipment, you can do those in your room at your convenience. Try to give yourself this important attention first thing in the morning, before other demands make themselves felt.

• Long plane flights make an ideal setting for a limited exercise routine—and a sorely needed one, too, if you are to avoid feeling cramped and stiff from too much sitting. Walk the aisles whenever the cabin crew allows. Try a few neck stretches in your seat.

• If you make long road trips in your car, do stop frequently to stretch and walk. These preventive measures can keep you from arriving at your destination in pain.

How to Modify Your Exercise Program During Illness

• Bad colds and flus will most likely ground you from your aerobic exercise. But you may be able to carry on with at least some of your stretching and strengthening in bed. And you may need to—if lying still for long periods of time leaves you stiff and uncomfortable.

• You may well find that stopping your aerobic exercise for any reason, for any period of time, actually leaves you feeling depressed. You've grown accustomed to the pleasant natural high you get when your heart and lungs are functioning at their peak performance, your muscles moving smoothly, and your brain releasing the body's own opiates, the endorphins. Promise yourself that you'll get back to regular walking or swimming as soon as your fever breaks.

P A R T
T H R E E

The Exercises

> All the step-by-step instructions
> are spelled out here, accompanied
> by line drawings to further clarify
> each exercise movement.

CHAPTER 8

Exercises for
Low-Back Pain

The exercises in this chapter focus on the site of most people's back pain. The word "low" is almost superfluous, because nearly everyone who has a backache has pain in the lower back. Right at the spot where you can reach around and place a comforting hand on your back at waist height—that's where the pain often starts.

The remedy is on the other side, in the muscles that run from the ribs to the pelvis—up and down, around, and through your torso. These abdominal muscles, which consist of several layers of interacting fibers, control your posture and body alignment. Weakness or injury in these muscles usually translates into back pain. It stands to reason, then, that strengthening the abdominal muscles (and thereby protecting

73

them from injury) can help prevent acute episodes of low-back pain. It's also true that gentle stretching of the lower back and strengthening of the abdominals can constitute a pain-relieving treatment for chronic low-back problems.

All of these exercises have been judged safe and effective for most people by the participants in our Back Pain Survey and by physician exercise specialists at The New York Hospital–Cornell University Medical Center. As with any exercise program, be sure to check with your doctor in case you have special restrictions. The exercises are grouped according to the important exercise goals of this chapter: stretching the lower back, strengthening the abdominal muscles, and stretching and strengthening the muscles of the buttocks, hips, and legs.

As you begin to exercise, listen to your body. You risk injury by pushing yourself through pain. The bodybuilder's adage, "No pain, no gain," simply doesn't apply here. In back exercise, the only important goal is normal function in everyday life. There's no one competing with you, so please don't push yourself too hard.

Start out with a maximum of three repetitions of each exercise you attempt. Advance slowly. Give yourself at least a week at each repetition level before you try to add more repetitions. And there's no point, really, in going beyond ten repetitions of any one exercise. Once you are strong and limber enough to work through ten repetitions of all the exercises in your program with ease, you can spend that much more time out walking or investigating other activities that bring you pleasure.

To Stretch the Lower Back

KNEES-TO-CHEST ROCK

This soft rocking motion takes advantage of the built-in relaxation of the knees-to-chest position. You will be giving yourself a slight lower-back massage in the process!

Starting position: Lie on your back, knees bent and feet flat on the floor, with your arms at your sides.

Steps:
1. Pull both knees to your chest, one at a time. (If you prefer, you may bring both knees up simultaneously.)
2. Hold your knees in this position. (For greatest ease, hold the backs of your thighs. If you are slightly more limber, hold your knees. To get the maximum stretch, clasp your arms around and just under both knees.)
3. Curl your head and shoulders forward, and gently rock to and fro, and from side to side in this position.

Note: Some people feel a strain in the neck while doing this exercise. If you feel just a slight strain with no pain afterward, there should be no reason to skip this one. But if it makes you genuinely uncomfortable, ease off until you have strengthened your neck with the exercises recommended for that purpose.

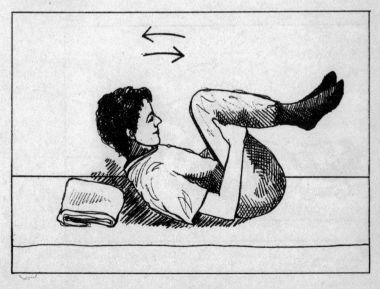

KNEE-TO-CHEST

As you lift your knee to your chest in this gentle stretch, you will feel the curve in your lower back flatten out.

Starting position: Lie on your back, knees bent and feet flat on the floor, arms relaxed at your sides.

Steps:
1. Lift your right knee toward your chest as far as you can. (For extra stretch, try pulling your knee a bit closer to your chest with your hands.) *a*
2. Lower that same knee to and through the starting position, so that your right leg is extended straight. *b*
3. Wobble your leg to relax your muscles. *c*
4. Return to the starting position.
5. Repeat steps 1–4 with your left leg.

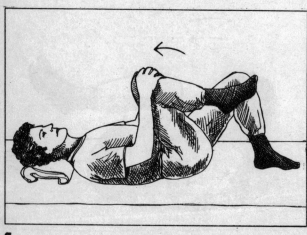

a

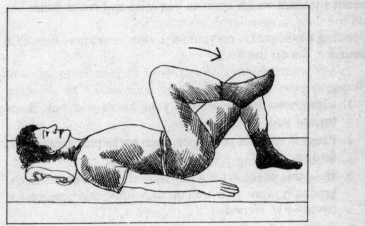

b

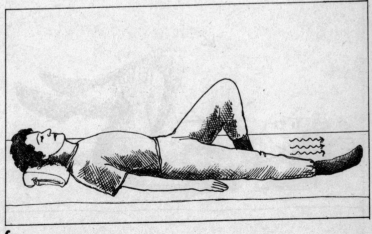

c

DOUBLE KNEE-TO-CHEST

The easiest way to perform this exercise is by keeping your knees together as you pull them to your chest. With experience, and for a greater stretch, you can try holding your knees about shoulder-width apart as you raise and lower them.

Starting position: Lie on your back with your knees bent and your feet flat on the floor.

Steps:
1. Clasp your hands around your knees and pull them toward your chest.
2. Pause if you feel resistance, then try to pull gently a bit farther.
3. Hold this position for a few seconds. (For added stretch, gradually work your way up to holding this position for twenty-five seconds.)
4. Return to the starting position.

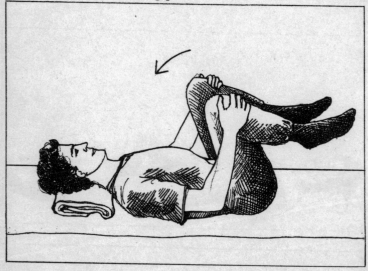

KNEE DROPS

Don't worry if you can't get your knees very far down when you first attempt this maneuver. You'll build up your ability in time.

Starting position: Lie on your back with your knees bent and your feet flat on the floor. *a*

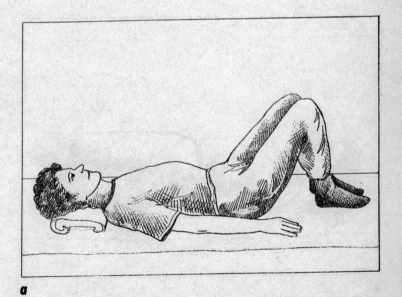

a

Steps:

1. Keeping your knees together, drop them both to the right as far as you can. (Your left hip and buttock will necessarily rise off the bed or floor as your knees drop to the right, but try to keep both your shoulders on the flat surface.) *b*
2. Return to the starting position. *c*
3. Drop both knees to the left. *d*

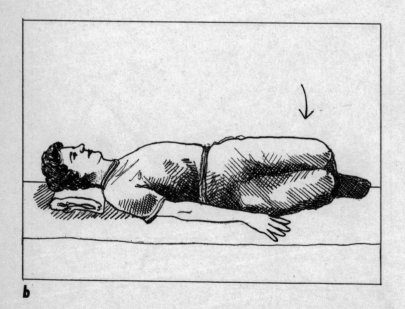

b

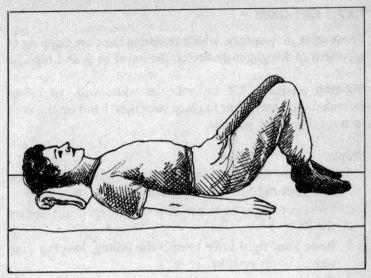

c

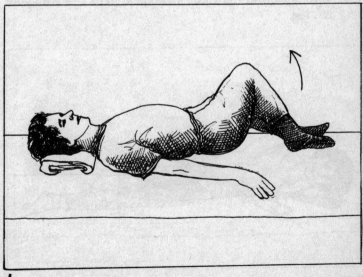

d

SIMPLE KNEE CROSS

These knee movements, which resemble the slow flapping of a butterfly's wing, gently stretch the lower back and hips.

Starting position: Lie on your left side, with your legs extended. You may want to place your right hand on the floor in front of you for support.

Steps:

1. Bend your right knee and pull it up toward your body so that your right foot is near your left knee. *a*
2. Press your right knee across your left leg, down toward the floor. *b*
3. Raise your right knee toward the ceiling, keeping your right foot on your left knee. *c*
4. Return to the starting position.
5. Turn onto your right side and repeat steps 1–4 with your left leg.

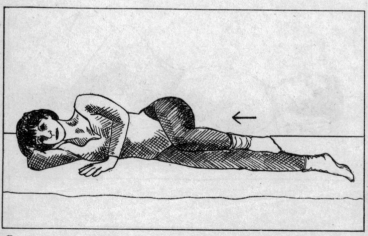

a

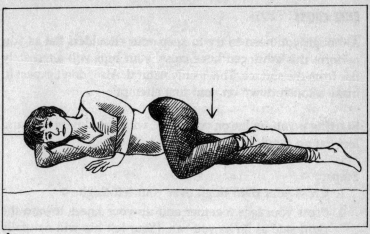

b

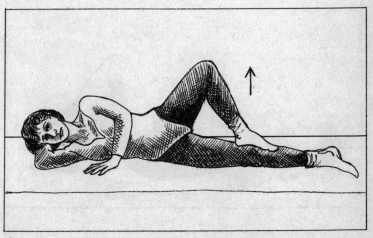

c

KNEE CROSS

Although you need to try to keep your shoulders flat as you perform this advanced knee cross, your hips will alternately rise from the surface. That's only natural. Also, don't expect to make a touch-down on your first attempt.

Starting position: Lie on your back, with your knees bent and feet flat on the floor, arms relaxed at your sides.

Steps:
1. Cross your right thigh over your left thigh. *a*
2. Press your legs together and tip your knees toward the right side as far as you can. (Your left hip will naturally rise as you do this.) *b*
3. Raise your knees and return to the starting position.
4. Repeat steps 1–3 on the other side, crossing your left thigh over the right, and tipping toward the left. *c*

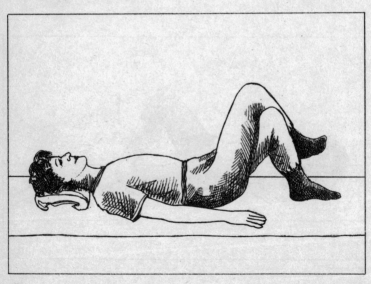

a

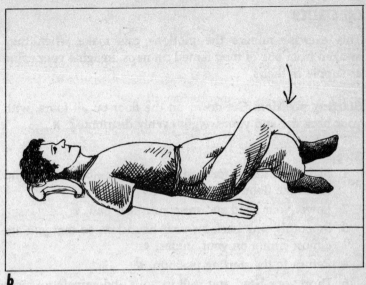

b

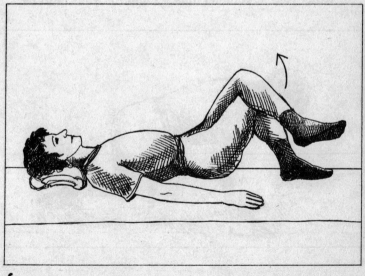

c

CAT STRETCH

This exercise mimics the motions cats make when they awaken from one of their famed cat naps. Imagine your spine as supple as theirs.

Starting position: Get down on the floor on all fours, with your back flat and your weight evenly distributed. *a*

Steps:
1. Slide your hands forward, letting your elbows bend and touch the floor.
2. Lower your head and raise your rear end. *b*
3. Smoothly sink back on your haunches, so that you are almost sitting on your ankles. *c*
4. Return to the starting position. *d*
5. Drop your head and pull in your abdominals to curve your back like a Halloween cat. *e*
6. Relax your abdominal muscles and roll your head back.

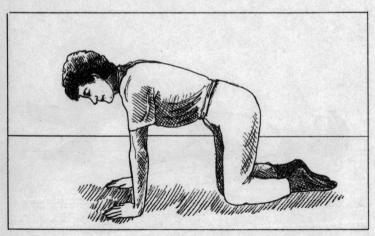

a

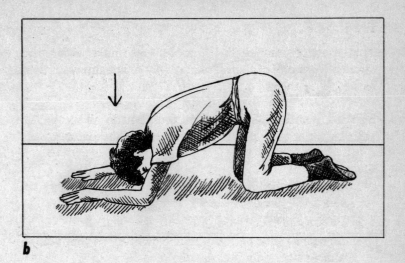

b

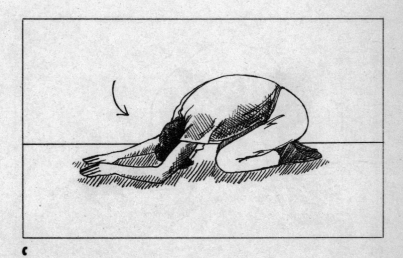

c

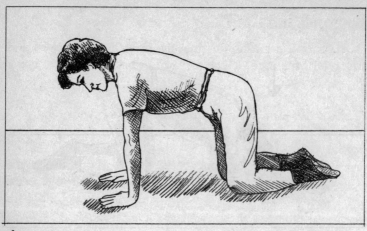

d

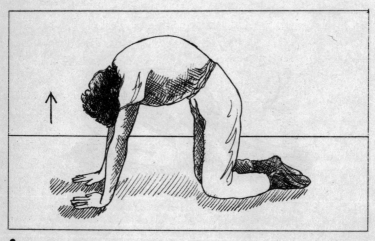

e

TWISTS AND TILTS

Give yourself a maximum sideways stretch as you twist and turn. Fight the urge to lean forward or backward, or to move your lower body.

Starting position: Stand with your hands on your hips.

Steps:
1. Lean the top of your body to the right. Resist the temptation to lean forward or backward as you bend sideways. Also try to keep your feet, legs, and hips steady. *a*
2. Straighten up slowly.
3. Repeat these motions to the left. *b*

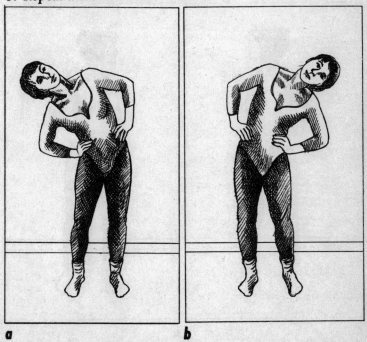

a   *b*

4. Twist the upper half of your body around to the left, as though you were trying to see behind you. **c**
5. Return to face front.
6. Repeat these motions to the right. **d**

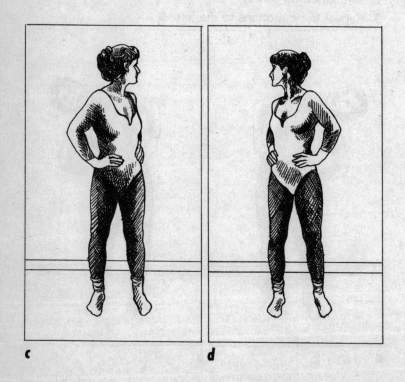

c   d

To Strengthen the Abdominal Muscles

PELVIC TILT

This most basic strengthening exercise will flatten both your abdomen and the curve in your lower back.

Starting position: Lie on your back with your knees bent and your feet flat on the floor, arms relaxed at your sides. *a*

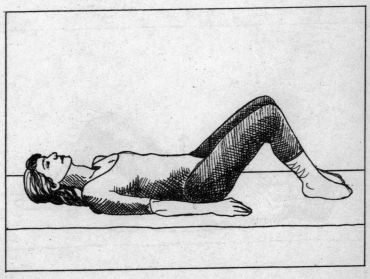

a

Steps:

1. Tighten your buttocks and pull in your abdominal muscles, so that your hips roll upward. Exhale as you do this. (Strive to work your buttocks and abdominal muscles, and resist the temptation to simply push off from the floor with your feet or hips.) *b*

2. Hold the position, but not your breath, for a few seconds.

3. Relax your muscles as you inhale and return to the starting position.

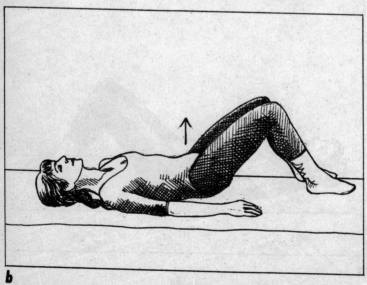

b

STANDING PELVIC TILT

A wall takes the place of bed or floor in this upright version of the basic Pelvic Tilt.

Starting position: Stand with your back against a wall, your feet a few inches out from the wall's base. *a*

Steps:
1. Exhaling, squeeze your buttocks together and pull in your gut, so that you can feel the curve in the small of your back flatten against the wall. Keep your shoulders relaxed as you do this. *b*
2. Hold the position for a few seconds as you breathe in and out normally.
3. Inhaling, relax and return to the starting position.

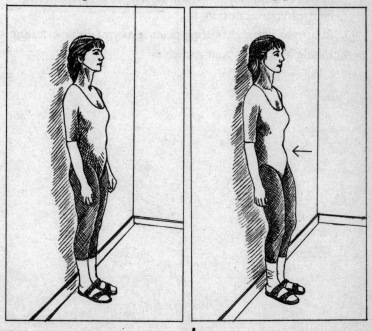

a   *b*

SIT-DOWNS

These reverse sit-ups are a bit more challenging, so please don't attempt them until you've built up your abdominal strength. Remember that the distance you move is secondary to the effort you put into strengthening your abdominal muscles.

Starting position: Sit on a bed or a bench that allows you room to lean back. Fold your arms across your chest. *a*

Steps:
1. Use your abdominal muscles to lean your body backward several inches—about as far as you would lift up for a sit-up. Exhale as you go. *b*
2. Hold the position, but don't hold your breath, for a count of three. Continue to exhale slowly, as this will help you control your abdominals.
3. Return to a straight sitting posture as you finish exhaling.
4. Inhale and relax your muscles.

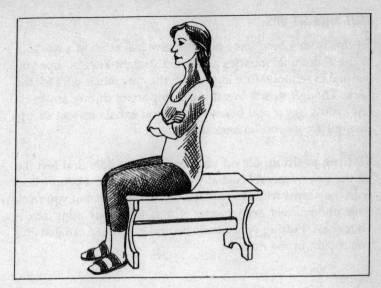

a

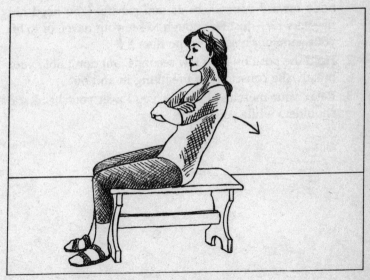

b

BENT-KNEE SIT-UPS

Sit-ups from a bent-knee position give just as good a workout to the abdominal muscles as the old straight-knee sit-ups you learned in school. More important, they are much safer for the back. Though steady breathing is important during any exercise, you'll get a real boost here if you exhale as you sit up, then inhale as you lie back down.

Starting position: Lie on your back, knees bent and feet flat on the floor, arms relaxed at your sides *(a)*. Most people lead with their arms when they perform this exercise, but you work your abdominals even harder if you fold your arms across your chest. Putting your hands behind your head can just give you a pain in the neck.

Steps:
1. Pull in your abdominals and raise the upper part of your body toward your knees as you exhale. (You need not rise very far—just far enough to see your navel, or to lift your shoulder blades off the floor.) *b*
2. Hold the position for a few seconds, but don't hold your breath. (Be conscious of breathing in and out.)
3. Relax your muscles slowly as you lower your head and shoulders while you inhale.

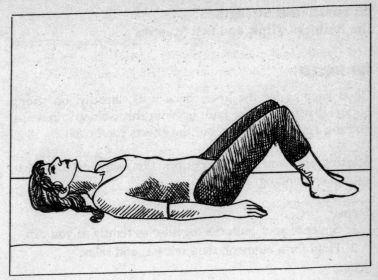

a

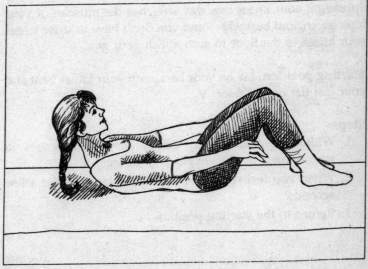

b

To Stretch and Strengthen the Buttocks, Hips, and Leg Muscles

THE SQUEEZE

Good support for the lower back rests, literally, on strong buttocks, which can be built up with this isometric exercise; nothing appears to move, but the effects can be felt.

Starting position: You may perform this exercise lying down, sitting, or standing.

Steps:
1. Squeeze your buttocks together as tightly as you can.
2. Hold for a moment, then release, and relax.

KNEE SPREAD

Spreading your knees this way stretches the muscles of your hips, groin, and buttocks—and you don't have to strive to get your knees to the floor to accomplish your goal.

Starting position: Lie on your back with your knees bent and your feet flat on the floor. *a*

Steps:
1. Without expending any effort, allow your knees to spread apart by the weight of your legs. *b*
2. When you feel resistance, hold your legs still for a few seconds.
3. Return to the starting position.

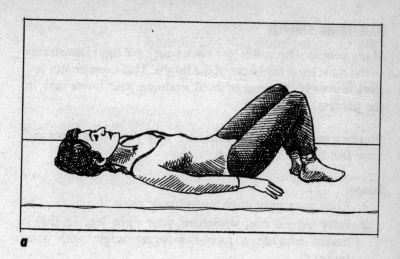

a

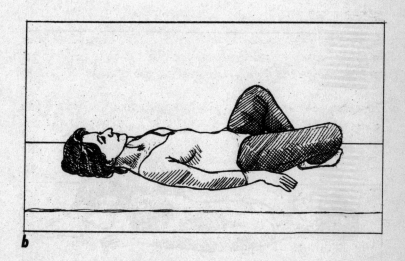

b

HAMSTRING STRETCH

Many people who suffer low-back pain have tight hamstrings —the muscles at the backs of the thighs. This exercise lets you stretch your hamstrings without straining your lower back in the process.

Starting position: Lie on your back with your knees bent and your feet flat on the floor. *a*

Steps:
1. Raise your right knee toward your chest. *b*
2. Fully extend and straighten your right leg, so that it makes roughly a forty-five-degree angle with your body. *c*

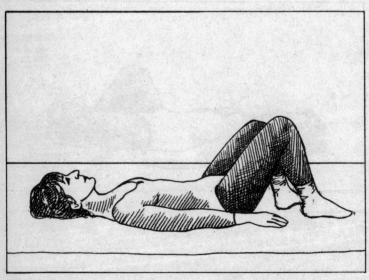

a

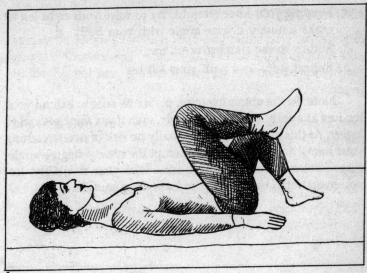

b

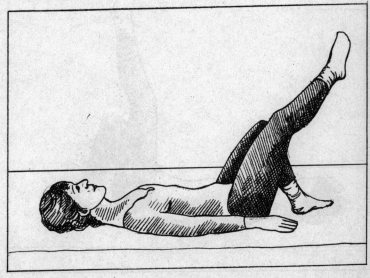

c

3. Keeping your knee straight, try to raise your right leg to make a ninety-degree angle with your body. *d*
4. Return to the starting position.
5. Repeat steps 1–4 with your left leg.

Note: In the above exercise, please be sure to extend your leg first at a forty-five-degree angle, *even if you think you can go higher*. At this angle, there is virtually no risk of overstretching your hamstrings. Before you attempt the ninety-degree angle, assure yourself that you have increased your flexibility, lest you overstretch or "pop" your hamstring muscle.

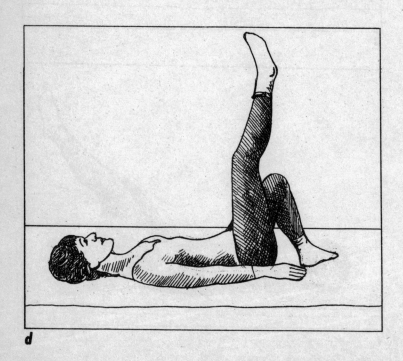

d

HIP HIKERS

Keeping full range of motion in your hips (a goal of this exercise) safeguards both your posture and your walking gait.

Starting position: Lie on your right side, with your knees straight and your right arm under your head. Prop your left hand on the floor in front of your body for support.

Steps:
1. Slowly lift your left leg as high as you can, keeping the knee straight.
2. Hold this extension for several seconds, feeling the stretch in your hip and thigh.
3. Gently lower your leg.
4. Repeat steps 1–3 twice. (This counts as three repetitions.)
5. Turn over and repeat the exercise, raising your right leg.

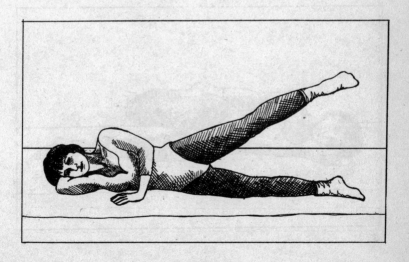

THIGH PULL

The flip side of the hamstrings are the quadriceps muscles at the front of the thighs. This exercise emphasizes body alignment as it stretches the area from hip to knee.

Starting position: Lie on your right side, your head resting on your right arm, and your left leg bent at the knee. Think of your body making a straight line from your head down the fronts of your thighs.

Steps:
1. With your left hand, grasp your left ankle. *a*
2. Keeping the knee bent, pull your left leg back and toward your buttocks as far as you comfortably can. Resist the temptation to arch your back.

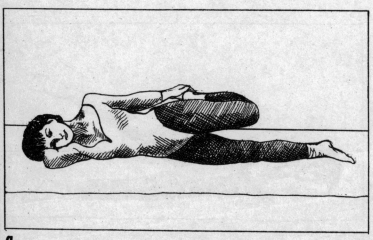

a

3. Hold this position for a few moments, feeling the stretch along the front of your thigh.
4. Return to the starting position.
5. Repeat steps 1–4 twice. *b*
6. Turn onto your left side, and repeat the exercise with your right leg.

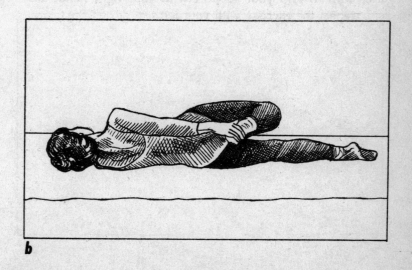

b

STANDING THIGH PULL

Holding your body in a Standing Pelvic Tilt while you do the following exercise will keep you properly aligned and help you avoid arching your back.

Starting position: Stand alongside a chair or other sturdy support that you can hold for balance.

Steps:
1. With your left hand on the support, bend your right knee and grasp your right ankle. *a*
2. Pull your right leg back and toward your buttocks, but not so far as to make you arch your back. *b*
3. Hold this position, feeling the stretch along the front of your thigh.
4. Release your ankle and slowly straighten your knee to return to the starting position.
5. Repeat steps 1–4 twice.
6. Turn to grip your support with your right hand, and repeat the exercise with your left leg.

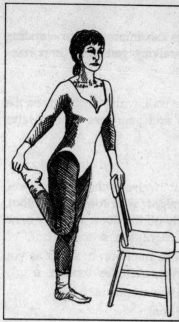

a

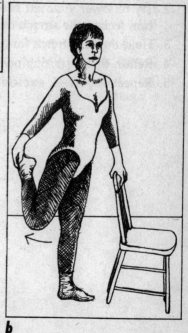

b

RUNNER'S STRETCH

Fully stretching your lower legs can improve your standing posture and smooth out your walking gait—two important factors in warding off back pain.

Starting position: Stand facing a wall, with your hands on the wall at about shoulder height, and your feet about twelve inches away from the wall's base.

Steps:
1. Extend your left leg about twelve inches behind you, keeping your left knee straight, your toes on the floor, and your heel raised slightly off the floor. You may bend the knee of your standing (right) leg. *a*
2. Try to lower your left heel to the floor, or as far as you can, feeling the stretch in your Achilles' tendon. *b*
3. Hold the full stretch for a few moments.
4. Return to the starting position.
5. Repeat steps 1–4, stretching your right leg.

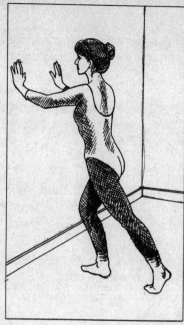

a

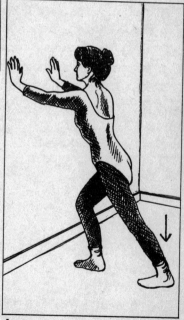

b

CHAPTER 9

Exercises for Upper-Back and Neck Pain

Although many doctors view upper-back and neck pain as "low-back pain that has migrated upward," different treatments and exercises apply.

In our original Back Pain Survey, less than half of the participants with neck pain were even aware that exercise could add strength and flexibility to their neck muscles. The other half—the participants with neck pain who did perform exercises to relieve that pain—saw improvement in their symptoms. The truth is, the results from neck exercise were not as dramatic as the results of exercise for low-back pain. But, based on our survey reports, we believe you can greatly improve your chances of getting a dramatic benefit from neck exercise by following a few simple guidelines:

• *Combine the neck exercises in this chapter with the low-back exercises in chapter 8.* Most of those survey participants with neck pain *also* had some pain or discomfort in the lower back. Performing both sets of exercises in a regular routine brought the most significant improvement.

• *Perform neck exercises frequently throughout the day.* Most of the movements described below can serve to relieve on-the-spot tension—as well as to build strength and flexibility. In other words, these exercises are "first aid" for neck pain. Any time you feel stress and discomfort accumulating in your neck, whether you are at work or at home, you may try alleviating the tension with a few neck exercises. Here, slight discomfort is expected while exercising. Remember, though, to drop any exercise that—*for you*—turns mild discomfort to pain.

• *Maintain good posture through your neck.* A mention of posture usually makes people suck in their abdominal muscles and throw their shoulders back. Since the spine begins in the neck, good posture also means keeping the head well aligned, as though it were a golden eagle on the top of a flagpole. To correct your neck posture, stretch your neck and head skyward momentarily—go straight up, as though your neck had grown longer—then relax and tuck in your chin, instead of letting it jut or droop. (See chapters 14 and 15 for more suggestions on maintaining proper alignment and avoiding neck pain during everyday activities such as reading or talking on the telephone.)

To Stretch the Neck

LEFT-RIGHT

These slow head turns to left and right help untie the knots of tension in the neck.

Starting position: You can do this exercise lying on your back in bed, or sitting or standing, with your arms at your sides.

Steps:

1. Keeping your head level, turn it to the right as far as you can, as though to stare across your right shoulder. *a*
2. Return your head and your gaze to center. *b*
3. Turn your head the other way to look as far left as you can.
4. Return to the starting position.

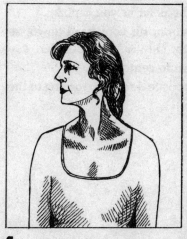
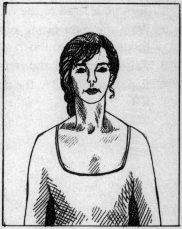

a   *b*

YES-NO

Nodding "yes" or shaking your head "no," the neck gets a workout by moving the head about.

Starting position: You may sit or stand virtually anywhere.

Steps:
1. Nod your head up and down slowly, several times.
2. Turn your head from side to side, as though making a slow, exaggerated "no" gesture.

LEFT-RIGHT PLUS

The extra chin-to-shoulder dip brings an added dimension to the side-to-side neck stretch.

Starting position: As above, you may lie on your back, or sit or stand with your arms at your sides. *a*

Steps:
1. Turn your head to the right as far as you can. *b*
2. From the right-facing position, tilt your head down, as though trying to touch your chin to your shoulder. *c*
3. Raise your head and return to center.
4. Repeat steps 1–3 in the opposite direction, turning to the left.

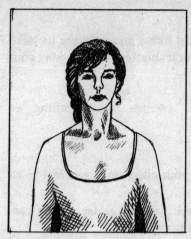

a

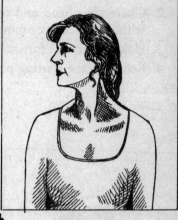

b

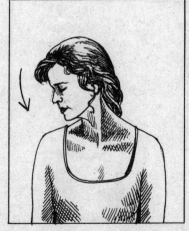

c

NECK BOB

This exercise may make you feel like a turtle poking its head out of its shell for a look-see, but it should also help relax your neck through a gentle stretch.

Starting position: Do this exercise while sitting or standing.

Steps:
1. Lower your chin toward your chest until you feel some resistance. *a*
2. Crane your head and neck forward as far as you can, without bending or moving your torso.
3. Hold the craned-forward position for a few seconds. *b*
4. Return to the starting position.

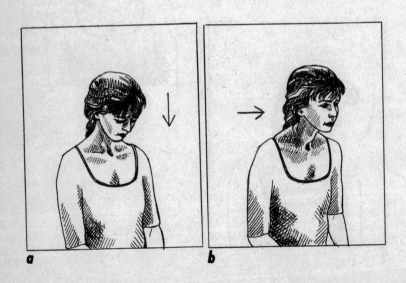

a   *b*

HEAD ROLL

This slow, continuous roll of the head gently stretches the neck muscles. You can make the side-to-side motions part of an in-bed exercise routine if you like. Remember, you get more of a stretch if you hold your shoulders still—and don't bring them up to meet your ears.

Starting position: Sit in a chair or stand at ease as you hold your head high and look straight ahead.

Steps:
1. Tilt your head to the left as though you were trying to put your ear on your shoulder. Stop when you've stretched your neck as far as you can. Don't try to bring your shoulder up to meet your ear. *a*
2. Roll your head forward and down, as though trying to touch your chin to your chest. *b*

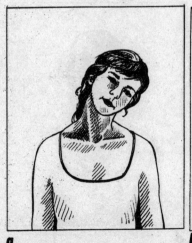
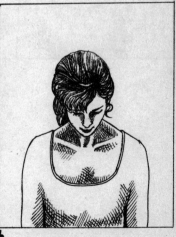

a   *b*

3. Continue the roll toward the right, as though trying to place your right ear on your right shoulder. **c**
4. Come full circle by tilting your head back, but not too far. (Feel free to omit this step, with its tilt backward, if arching is a problem for your upper spine.) **d**
5. Return to the starting position.
6. Repeat steps 1–5 in the opposite direction, circling your head to the left this time.

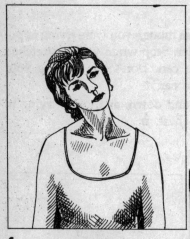

c

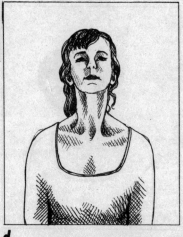

d

HEAD PULL

You may be able to get the most stretch in your neck by pulling your head with your hands.

Starting position: Sit in a chair with your back straight and your hands clasped behind your head. *a*

Steps:
1. Gently pull your head forward and down to stretch the back of your neck. *b*
2. Hold, feeling the stretch.
3. Return to the starting position.

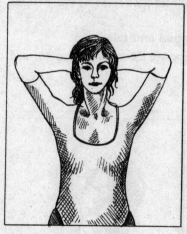

a

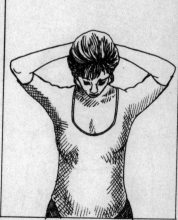

b

NECK TILT

Instead of a continuous rolling motion, this sideways neck stretch calls to mind the motions of an attentive bird, cocking its head first one way, then the other.

Starting position: Sit or stand comfortably, facing straight ahead.

Steps:
1. Tilt your head to the left, as though trying to touch your ear to your shoulder. Don't try to bring your shoulder up to your ear. *a*
2. When you feel resistance, pause for a few seconds to hold the position.
3. Return to the starting position and relax.
4. Repeat steps 1–3 in the opposite direction, tilting toward the right. *b*

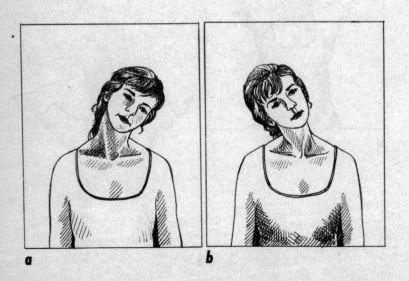

a   *b*

To Strengthen the Neck

BED HEAD

Your head makes a handy weight for your neck to press and push in this strengthening exercise.

Starting position: Lie on your back in bed or on the floor.

Steps:
1. Press your head straight back into your pillow or mat.
2. Hold for a moment, then release the pressure.
3. Lift your head above your pillow or mat as high as you can, without lifting your shoulders.
4. Hold, feeling the effort in your neck, then release.

NECK PUSH

This isometric exercise can strengthen your neck by making it work against the pressure of your own arm strength. You can also try doing it by pressing your forehead against a wall!

Starting position: Sit or stand comfortably, arms at your sides.

Steps:
1. Press the palm of one hand against your forehead, and your forehead against the palm of your hand.
2. Hold for a moment, keeping the pressure on your hand and head without moving either one.
3. Relax and return to the starting position.

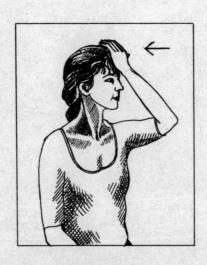

SIDE NECK PUSH

The hand-on-head stance called for here may imitate a look of anguish, but the results should bring relief instead.

Starting position: Do this exercise sitting, standing, or even lying down, arms at your sides.

Steps:
1. Press your left hand against the left side of your head, and simultaneously press your head against your hand.
2. Hold the position, hand and head pushing against each other.
3. Relax and return to the starting position.
4. Repeat steps 1–3, raising your right hand to the right side of your head.

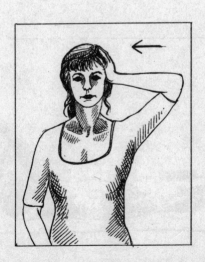

To Stretch the Shoulders and Upper Back

PRONE SHOULDER STRETCH

Try not to raise your shoulders in this exercise, but just let the flowing motion of your arm stretch the neck and shoulder muscles.

Starting position: Lie on your back with your knees bent and feet flat, arms at your sides.

Steps:
1. Raise your right arm straight up to a ninety-degree angle, and keep moving it through a half-circle until it is extended behind you, palm up.
2. Relax for a moment, and then reverse movement and return to the starting position.
3. Repeat steps 1 and 2 with your left arm.

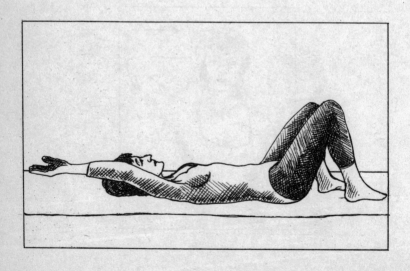

SHOULDER SHRUG

Even though your shoulders do the work by shrugging, your neck will appear to shrink and grow—and feel the positive effects over time.

Starting position: You can do this exercise lying in bed or sitting or standing, with your arms at your sides.

Steps:
1. Slowly and steadily raise your shoulders to a shrug. *a*
2. Hold for a moment, feeling the effect on your neck muscles.
3. Keeping your head still, gently press your shoulders as far down as you can. *b*
4. Hold, feeling the stretch in your neck.

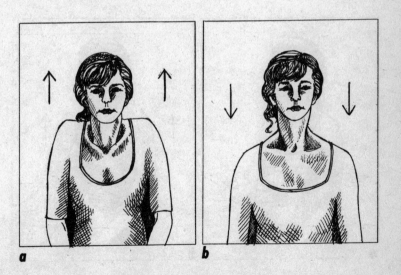

a   *b*

SHOULDER ROLL

Try to roll your shoulders through a full circle in one fluid motion. Even though each step is numbered separately, keep moving slowly from one to the next without stopping.

Starting position: Sit or stand with your shoulders relaxed. *a*

Steps:
1. Raise your shoulders. *b*
2. Bring your shoulders forward. *c*
3. Push your shoulders down. *d*
4. Pull your shoulders back. *e*
5. Return to the starting position. *f*
6. Circle your shoulders in the opposite direction, reversing the order of steps 1–5.

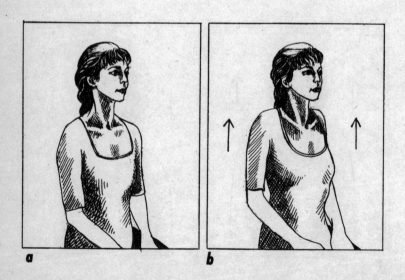

a   b

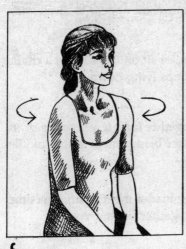

c

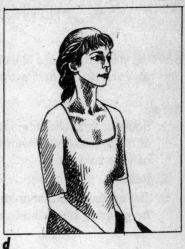

d

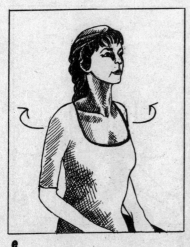

e

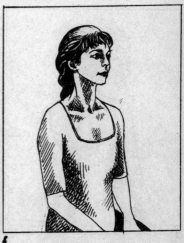

f

ROLLER BLADES

This rolling movement of the shoulder blades feels like a sideways shrug. It will make your chest appear to swell with pride.

Starting position: Stand at ease, or sit on the edge of a chair. You can even do the first two steps lying down.

Steps:
1. Squeeze your shoulders together for a few seconds in an effort to make your shoulder blades meet in the middle of your back. *a*
2. Relax.
3. Try to make your shoulder blades meet again, this time by pushing your elbows together behind you. *b*

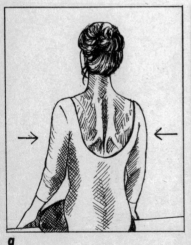
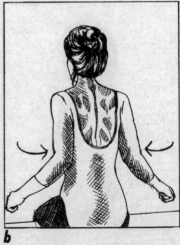

a

b

SQUARE SHOULDER STRETCH

Try to keep your neck relaxed as one arm pulls the other to stretch the deltoid muscles of your shoulders and upper arms.

Starting position: Sit on a straight-backed chair or stool. Cross your arms in front of you, left over right, so that each hand holds the opposite elbow, raise your arms over your head in this way, and then let your left hand hang free. *a*

Steps:
1. With your right hand, pull your left elbow toward and behind your head. *b*
2. Hold this stretch for several seconds, feeling the stretch in your shoulder and upper arm.
3. Relax and return to the starting position, and switch your grip to hold your right elbow in your left hand.
4. Repeat steps 1–3, using your left hand to pull your right elbow.

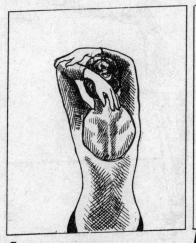
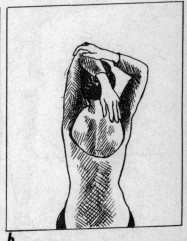

a   *b*

AIRPLANE

Try to keep your neck relaxed and your posture aligned as you make these motions of a child imitating an airplane.

Starting position: Stand with your arms straight out to the sides at shoulder height, palms down.

Steps:
1. Make several small forward circles with your arms, keeping your elbows straight.
2. Circle your arms in reverse.

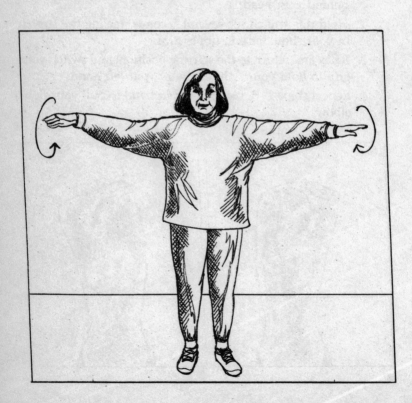

WINDMILL

Picture your arms as the blades of a windmill as you perform this exercise—but don't try to go as fast!

Starting position: Stand at ease, arms at your sides.

Steps:
1. Keeping your right arm straight, describe several huge circles in the air in a forward motion. *a b*
2. Without stopping, circle your right arm in the opposite direction, going through a full range of motion.
3. Repeat steps 1–3 with your left arm.

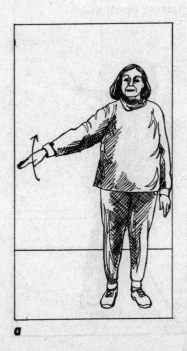 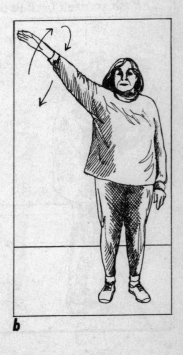

a   *b*

To Strengthen the Shoulders and Upper Back

PUSH-OFFS

These standing push-ups are easier than the military kind. They increase in difficulty as you increase the distance between yourself and the wall to as far as two feet.

Starting position: Stand facing a wall, with your feet apart and about twelve inches away from the wall, with your palms resting on the wall at shoulder height. *a*

Steps:
1. Lean in toward the wall as far as possible, keeping your legs and back straight. *b*
2. Push yourself back to the starting position.

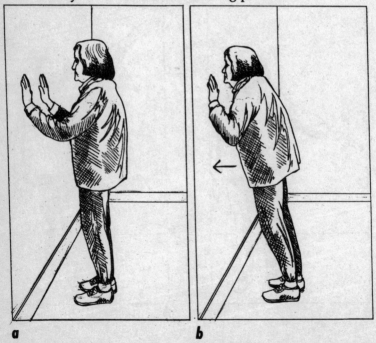

a   *b*

SIDE PRESS

Stubbornly pushing against a wall is a sound isometric approach to increasing shoulder strength.

Starting position: Stand near a wall, with the left side of your body about six inches away from it.

Steps:
1. Extend your left arm out sideways until your forearm is pressing against the wall. *a*
2. Continue to push for several seconds, feeling the exertion in your shoulder.

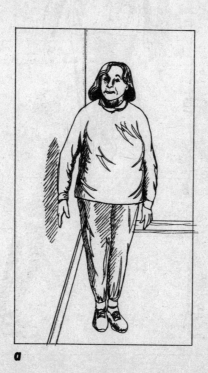

a

3. Relax and return to the starting position.
4. Repeat steps 1–3 twice. *b*
5. Turn, and repeat the exercise with your right arm.

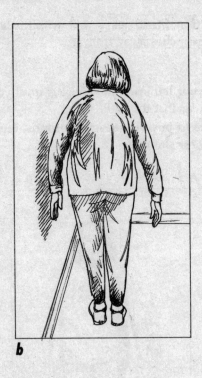

b

CHAPTER 10

Exercises for General Fitness

Fitness has become such a popular national pursuit that you can barely walk down the street these days without encountering joggers, cyclists, and rollerbladers out in force. But if you are walking down the street, you are already engaged in the all-time best activity for building cardiovascular fitness and keeping your back limber.

In this chapter we'll be discussing the four most popular fitness exercises for people with back pain—walking, swimming, cycling, and dancing.

Walking

Walking is the oldest and best of the weight-bearing exercises for people with back pain. Walking proved helpful in the long run for 98 percent of the participants in our Back Pain Survey who made this activity a regular part of their routine. They reported that walking not only increased the flexibility of their backs, but also improved their overall strength and muscle tone. Another important advantage was that walking at least thirty minutes a day, four times a week, greatly reduced stress and tension for these people. Even the twenty-six participants who couldn't lead normal lives because of back pain *all* improved in the long run by following their practitioners' advice to walk (or swim) regularly.

Hospital studies show that walkers accrue the same cardiovascular benefits that runners do, and with far fewer injuries. It makes an ideal back exercise because it is low-impact yet high-endurance—that is, once you have built up to taking relatively long walks several times a week. Because most people can walk for a longer time than they can run or play tennis, for example, walking tends to build muscular endurance while it burns calories.

Walking is easy, accessible, effective, and enjoyable. It can be geared to any level of fitness, and pursued by people of all ages. No exercise could be more convenient than walking. You need no special equipment and no special clothing, other than comfortable shoes. You don't have to travel to the gym or the pool; you just get up and go. For these reasons, you're far less likely to quit your walking regimen than any other exercise you might try.

Most people can easily fit walking into their daily activities if they try. You may even find that you can combine your daily activities—your errands, some light shopping—with your walk when you are pressed for time. Walking to work or to appointments is another way to fit exercise into the day's program. And although walking will quicken your heart rate and get your body into condition, it typically doesn't leave you perspiring so much that you require a shower or a change of clothing when you get where you're going.

If you are already in reasonably good shape, we recommend at least half an hour of brisk walking every other day. You may build up to walking three or four miles in an hour, five to seven days a week. What starts out as something you do to improve your back may well turn into the highlight of your day—the time you feel simultaneously relaxed and energized. At that point, you probably won't want to miss your daily walk.

Your walking pace is a measure of your fitness and freedom from pain. An ideal pace, according to Dr. James Rippe, director of the Exercise Physiology and Nutrition Laboratory at the University of Massachusetts School of Medicine, is to walk as though you have someplace to go. But Dr. John Duncan of the Cooper Institute for Aerobics Research in Dallas has shown in studies that even a slow pace can benefit your heart and lower your cholesterol level.

Most important, as far as your back is concerned, is to keep your posture alignment in check, with your abdominals holding your lower back in proper position. And walk with zest—with your hips and legs making great strides as you swing your arms and get the maximum enjoyment out of the activity.

At the risk of overstating the obvious, we would like to emphasize that the goal of walking is to move forward. Many people add extraneous motions to their walking gait. They may flop from side to side, or bounce up and down as they go. We want you to walk with your posture and purpose in mind. Try to imagine that you are being pulled forward by a string attached to the middle of your chest.

If you are just recuperating from an episode of incapacitating back pain, then you'll want to build up gradually to a fitness level of walking. You can begin by walking as much as you can around your house, as soon as you feel up to it. Even though you stay indoors, we urge you to wear good shoes as soon as you make the transition from being in bed most of the time to being up and about. A pair of walking or running shoes, or any comfortable shoes that offer good support, will help you through this recovery period. The best shoes are those you're already used to. If you do need to break in a new pair of shoes, we urge you to do it gradually, because any sudden change at this point could aggravate your back. (Even after you're up and about, we recommend wearing new shoes just half an hour the first time, then an additional half hour each succeeding day.)

When you venture outside the first few times, try to avoid steep grades and uneven ground, as walking up or down hills causes more of a strain on the muscles of the lower back. What's more, rocky ground or broken sidewalks can make it difficult for you to relax and stride comfortably, with your head held high and your gaze out to the world.

Swimming

Swimming is an ideal aerobic exercise for general fitness because it makes the arms and legs work hard to get the heart pumping. Some exercise experts, however, argue that swimming can't match up to walking or running as a weight-bearing exercise. Although it's true that the water provides a virtually stress-free environment, studies have shown that swimmers have thicker, stronger bones than people who perform no exercise at all. Swimming can indeed help you improve your muscle endurance and flexibility.

We didn't hear a single negative comment about swimming in our Back Pain Survey. We did, however, hear a few cautionary notes about which stroke to choose. A tiring, taxing stroke such as the butterfly, for example, which requires the arms to whirl like windmills while the lower back and legs mimic a leaping dolphin, is clearly too risky for anyone with back problems.

Some people with back pain find that the standard overhand crawl or "freestyle" puts too much of an arch in the lower back. Many prefer the sidestroke, with its froglike kicking motions, to the back-arching flutter-kick of the crawl. We consider the sidestroke to be the easiest on the back, and we recommend that you alternate sides so that you exercise your body evenly. The backstroke—not the back crawl, but the breaststroke flipped on its back—is the next easiest. Keep it simple by keeping your arms close to your sides as you cup your hands to push through the water, instead of reaching way up beyond your shoulder level for power strokes. You may add a frog-kick or a flutter-kick—whichever feels better to you.

You can experiment with different strokes to find the one that suits you best. You may find you like to combine a variety of strokes to add interest to your time in the water. By alternating between difficult and simple strokes, you can pace yourself—getting a good workout while avoiding rapid fatigue.

One advantage of swimming over other fitness activities is that water makes exercise a virtually no-sweat proposition. The reason? Water is four times more efficient than air at dissipating heat. This keeps your body from getting overheated so quickly, and enables you to continue feeling comfortable even though you may be working out very hard in hot weather.

If you have a pool near you and can swim regularly, try to build up to fifteen minutes of nonstop swimming, three times a week. You may find that swimming is more beneficial to you than anything else, even walking, depending on your particular condition. (See chapter 11 for a full discussion of exercises for various back ailments.)

Bicycling

A bicycle may be your best friend or your worst enemy, depending on the way it requires you to sit, position your hands, and extend your neck. The racing bike, which asks the rider to assume a near-fetal position and then crane his or her neck up to see straight ahead, has at last given way in popularity to the upright touring and all-terrain or "mountain" bikes. This trend is a real boon to back sufferers. You will be much more comfortable sitting straight up than hunching over for the sake of reducing air resistance on your body. After all, when your purpose in riding is to gain exercise and fresh air, as opposed to winning a race, sitting up is the position of choice.

Seat comfort is an all-important consideration. Whether you ride as an excuse to get out and about, or restrict your pedaling to an indoor exercise bike, you need to remain seated throughout your workout. Some people experience nothing more annoying than a mild soreness in their buttocks the first few days of getting used to a bicycle seat. Others find that the pain never goes away. This is especially important for people with sciatica pain, which typically runs through the buttocks. Obviously, if you can't get comfortable on a bicycle, then cycling is not for you. But before you give up the advantages of this sport, try experimenting with comfort solutions. You can, for example, add a padded seat cover, or change the seat altogether. Most people find the broad "saddle" style more comfortable than the small, hard racing seat.

Since we are recommending bicycle riding as a good fitness activity, we must add that biking requires certain safety precautions that have nothing to do with posture or seat selection. Now that the pattern of bicycle-related injuries has been well documented, we urge you to buy and wear a bike helmet. Even top pros who rarely fall off a bicycle avow that head protection is essential on every ride—not only on streets shared with auto traffic, but also on special bicycle paths in parks. If you're a night rider, you'll need reflectors on your bicycle as well as on your clothing and helmet, for safety's sake. It's also a good idea to equip your bicycle with a headlight and taillight.

Cycling can be enjoyed as an indoor sport with a stationary exercise bike. Many busy people like to work out with an exercise bike, rooted to the floor, because it allows them to pedal away while getting something else done—reading a book or a magazine, say, watching television, or even viewing a movie on videocassette.

We tend to think of cycling as legwork, and it is, but some stationary bikes include activities for the arms, too. As you pump the pedals with your feet on one of these, you can push and pull handles that exercise your upper body.

Dancing

Health experts consider dancing a reasonable alternative to other aerobic activities, including walking, swimming, and cycling. As the most social of all these outlets, dancing provides the combination of good movements and good times with others that puts you in the swing of things and makes you feel good to be alive.

Ballroom dancing and folk dancing may offer just the right activity level for you, as they need not be stressful exercises. If your back is basically strong, causing you only minor aches and pain, you may choose to investigate modern dance, jazz, or even ballet instruction.

When you and your partner dance to the music of a long song set, continuing until the music ends, you get great endurance exercise. What's more, the chance to be with other people in an active form of recreation makes dancing virtually boredom-proof. People may abandon their exercise bikes and find excuses to avoid the swimming pool on a chilly day, but dancing retains its appeal over the long haul. It's one of the most enjoyable ways to rediscover how much your body can do.

One of the chief benefits of dancing is the relaxed style of movement that comes from mastering steps to music. If you take up dancing, you may well find that as you become accustomed to rhythmically positioning your body in space, you develop dancelike ways of doing other activities. Your motions may become more fluid, so that you improve your walking gait, for example. Instead of striking a rigid pose while you stand at the kitchen counter or sit at your desk, you may bring the good body mechanics of dancing to bear by adding a little motion. Some dancers gently dip and shift their weight from one leg to the other while working standing up, or perform a rock-and-roll stretch of the lower back while typing at the computer keyboard.

Several participants in our Back Pain Survey learned exercise from dance instructors who taught modern dance and ballet. They went for instruction after a painful episode had ended, not in the throes of back pain. They enjoyed the idea of learning to dance and of practicing at least three times a week. Most found they experienced substantial improvement in their posture, abdominal strength, and overall flexibility, along with a substantial reduction of back pain.

Some Asian martial arts, such as t'ai chi ch'uan, offer a non-jarring, dancelike form of aerobic exercise that can be practiced daily, by oneself or in a group.

CHAPTER 11

Exercises for Specific Conditions

When we talk about tailoring a back-exercise program to your specific needs, we have in mind the specific condition— provided that one can be identified—that is the root cause of your back pain. Many, if not most, back problems elude specific diagnoses agreed on by different kinds of practitioners. Some conditions, however, are easily recognized. And according to the results of our Back Pain Survey, exercises that take these back problems into account offer the best chance of improvement. Whether or not you can name your condition, you may still be able to categorize your back problem according to the nature of your pain, the type of situation that may aggravate your pain, and the area of your back that hurts most.

Please don't feel at a disadvantage if you can't rattle off a bona fide medical term such as "herniated disk" or "scoliosis" that neatly pigeonholes your backache. Hardly anyone knows such things for certain. We found that more than half of our original survey respondents had received two or more different diagnoses from two or more practitioners. Most of these discrepancies represented major differences of opinion—not just variations in terminology.

The good news is that even if you never find out exactly what's wrong with your back, you can still get well. After all, you do know your own symptoms, and that knowledge will help you "categorize" your own pain, so long as serious medical conditions have been ruled out as the cause of your pain.

Following is a list of what we have found to be the seven most common categories of back pain (for obvious reasons, some of the names sound more specific than others):

- low back
- herniated (ruptured) and degenerative disk
- neck
- osteoarthritis
- sciatica
- scoliosis
- spondylolisthesis

You may be able to place yourself in one of the above categories, or you may feel that you belong in two or more of them. Indeed, if you have a herniated disk, you may well have sciatica as a result. Low-back and neck pain are frequent companions. And osteoarthritis may superimpose itself on one or more existing back problems.

144

The rest of this chapter will look at these categories one by one, and offer specific exercise suggestions. According to our survey results, for example, bicycling turns out to be an excellent workout for people with scoliosis. If your back pain falls into more than one category, you'll find more than one section of this chapter of value.

Low Back

This is the leading cause of disability among American adults under age forty-five. Only colds and sore throats top low-back pain as reasons for seeking medical attention.

Whether you have recently been laid up with an acute case of low-back pain, or have a chronic painful condition, you can begin to address your needs with the "Basic Preparation" exercises outlined in chapter 6. These will help you make the transition from bed rest to restored normal activity.

The part of your exercise routine that brings you the most pleasure will likely be the stretching exercises. By easing the tendency to muscle spasm in your lower back, you will also be helping yourself prevent future pain and disability by faithfully performing your low-back stretches.

As you recuperate, try to walk as much as you can. Although you may be tempted at first to switch your environment from your bed to a chair, you'll no doubt find that sitting puts much more strain on your back than lying down or standing up. Keep walking. Try to walk at least two miles a day. Other people may get in enough walking on their jobs, but this may not be enough to control your low-back pain. You will really benefit from daily periods spent in brisk, mind-clearing, arm-swinging, uninterrupted walking.

Herniated (Ruptured) and Degenerative Disk

While suffering the intense pain of a herniated disk, you may well need to spend several weeks in bed as an alternative to surgery. Or you may have an operation and go through a lengthy recovery period.

Results from our Back Pain Survey suggest that people with herniated disks need to be especially careful about exercise, since their rate of exercise-related injury is high. Among our participants, 15 percent of those who had disk problems incurred injury from exercise, while only 3 percent of the participants with low-back pain found exercise harmful. The point, however, is not to avoid back exercises, but to know which exercises to do and when to do them.

Some specialists and some exercise books offer dangerous exercise advice, such as telling individuals to stretch their hamstrings by bending over and touching their toes. We consider this a formula for disaster. Double leg raises probably should be outlawed because of the pressure they put on the disks. The same is true for straight-leg sit-ups.

For you, building strength, especially in your abdominal muscles, takes priority over all stretching exercises. As general fitness exercises, nothing can beat walking and swimming. Try to pursue them both, beginning as soon as possible after your acute pain ebbs. Indeed, we urge you to begin putting your fitness program into effect as soon as you're out of bed. This measure will help you beat the odds of remaining limited by disability.

The best professional treatment for chronic ruptured-disk pain, as revealed in our survey, is individualized back-exercise therapy. If you have not been able to perform back exercises because of pain, don't quit yet. Please show the program in this book to your doctor. It is probably sufficient to put you on the track toward wellness, but don't hesitate to seek the personal advice of a physiatrist, physical therapist, or other expert instructor in exercise as rehabilitation.

Neck

Although neck pain is often viewed as a back problem that just happened to land higher up on the spine, the causes and treatments differ substantially. For example, low-back pain usually benefits from a few days of bed rest; neck pain hardly ever does. Unless the neck pain stems from a serious accident involving a car crash or a bad fall, bed rest may make it worse. According to the results of our Back Pain Survey, neck pain was more likely than any other variety of back pain to benefit from chiropractic care.

Our survey participants found that no single approach was sufficient to provide long-term help. Chronic neck-pain sufferers who did away with disabling pain found the success lay in a combination of exercise, posture adjustment, and stress reduction (often achieved through exercise).

Rarely does a person with neck pain require exercise instruction from a professional. Neck-saving maneuvers can be learned in a matter of minutes. Unfortunately, many people with neck pain miss out on the benefits of exercise simply because they don't think to do it. They may see the value of exercising their arms and legs, but they seem to put their necks in a different category. The truth is, neck exercises offer proven help for pain and stiffness. We encourage you to incorporate the neck exercises outlined in chapter 9 in your daily routine.

The objective of neck exercise is to promote relaxation, to stretch the neck muscles so as to make them more flexible, and to strengthen them. Our survey participants found they tended to perform neck exercises more frequently when they were experiencing some discomfort. In other words, these particular movements seem to provide on-the-spot relief.

Osteoarthritis

Signs of osteoarthritis—pain and stiffness in the joints of the spine, bony growths or spurs that show up on X rays—seem to multiply with age. Other forms of arthritis, however, including rheumatoid arthritis and ankylosing spondylitis, are found just as often among young adults as among older ones, and follow a completely different course.

Osteoarthritis is often called a "wear and tear" condition because the cartilage that protects the ends of the bones flakes off, leaving rough edges that prevent the joints from functioning smoothly. One of the reasons that exercise figures so importantly in arthritis treatment is that it helps nourish the joints, to slow or reverse their destruction. Motion squeezes fluids in and out of the joint spaces, facilitating the delivery of nutrients to the cartilage, which has no blood supply of its own, and the removal of waste products.

Rest, which was long touted as the best treatment for arthritis of any kind, has proved to be a poor and even destructive substitute for activity.

Stretching exercises, which are often called "range of motion" maneuvers by arthritis specialists, actually preserve the motion of the various joints. Coupled with strengthening exercises, they help protect the joints from injury by building a strong support network in the surrounding muscles, tendons, and ligaments. All of the exercises in chapters 8 and 9 are suitable for people with back pain resulting from osteoarthritis.

You may find that exercise improves your function even

more than it relieves your pain, though it often serves both purposes equally well.

Walking and swimming were the two fitness exercises that gave the greatest help to the participants in our Back Pain Survey who suffered from osteoarthritis. (We also conducted a separate Arthritis Survey, to uncover useful information for people with osteoarthritis and rheumatoid arthritis—not solely in the back, but in all the joints of the body.)

Sciatica

Knifelike pain that runs along the sciatic nerve may result from disk problems, osteoarthritis, or other, perhaps unidentified, causes. Often compared to a bad toothache of the body, sciatica typically begins in the buttocks, near the spot where the sciatic nerve emerges from the spinal column, then courses through the thigh and calf, and on into the foot.

Participants in our Back Pain Survey who suffered from sciatica were typically treated with drugs and surgery, but the ones who fared best made progress through prescribed exercise taught to them by physiatrists, physical therapists, and, in some cases, chiropractors.

Some of the best movements for sciatica prove to be Pelvic Tilts, mild stretches of the lower back, and a fitness concentration on swimming or walking. We want you to proceed with more than usual caution, since the risk of exercise-related injury in sciatica is comparable to that associated with herniated disk. It is all too easy to feel worse instead of better.

The exercises in chapter 8 make up the kind of safe-not-sorry program that can lead you to meaningful improvement in a few months' time.

Scoliosis

Unlike other participants in our Back Pain Survey, people with the spine curvature called scoliosis had better luck exercising without professional input. What's more, they fared better with fitness exercises than with the traditional stretching and strengthening movements. This may be because the spine can become rigid in scoliosis. Thus, a low-back stretch may not achieve for you what it achieves for a person with low-back pain. It may even be painful or awkward for you to lie flat on the floor in basic exercise positions, if your curvature makes one side of your back protrude beyond the other. And yet you can benefit enormously from exercises that keep you in motion—especially bicycling, swimming, and walking.

Our participants with scoliosis had nothing but praise for yoga as an exercise technique. Practicing yoga with an instructor who selected appropriate positions brought dramatic pain relief and a heightened sense of well-being.

The best scenario for people with scoliosis was to pursue, actively and regularly, a combination of two fitness activities, such as yoga and swimming.

We advise you to try the exercises in chapters 8 and 9, as we feel they can do no harm. But the more important advice for you is contained in chapter 10.

Spondylolisthesis

Many people have never even heard of this condition, which involves an actual slippage of one or more of the vertebrae, most often the lowest lumbar vertebra. The term "slipped disk," as we mentioned earlier, is a misnomer, as disks do not slip. Unfortunately, vertebrae *can* slip, causing great strain on the back muscles, as well as nerve compression and sciatica.

Only ten of the participants in our Back Pain Survey had a diagnosis of spondylolisthesis. Seven of them attributed their improved functioning and their pain relief to exercise, and a few mentioned yoga specifically as the form of exercise they favored. Proper exercise can actually stop the progression of this condition.

If you have spondylolisthesis, you can use the exercises in chapter 8 to strengthen your abdominal muscles, as this is one of the most important remedies. Walking and swimming are the safest fitness activities to include in your regimen.

P A R T
F O U R

Mind-Body Work

Mental exercises that promote
stress reduction and relaxation can
complement any physical exercise
program.

CHAPTER 12

Yoga

With its traditional emphasis on the integration of spine, mind, and spirit, yoga provides an excellent format for backache relief. In fact, our Back Pain Survey revealed yoga instruction and practice to be among the most successful of all treatment modalities for people who were not incapacitated by their back pain. And those participants who were troubled by osteoarthritis, neck pain, and scoliosis found it particularly effective.

The word *yoga* means "unity" or "harmony." Yoga is a way of healing the body through exercises that combine postures, movements, and breathing techniques.

To the extent that stretching and strengthening your body is helpful—and we believe this beyond a doubt—yoga instruction can be an excellent way to rid yourself of back pain. To the extent that stress contributes to back pain—and *most* of our survey participants felt that it did—yoga instruction can bring significant relief. The yoga philosophy of never forcing or straining, and of moving in a fluid, meditative manner, makes excellent sense for people with back problems. But yoga philosophy also encompasses the harmony of mind, body, and spirit—a concept that is difficult for some back sufferers to grasp, or to take seriously. Although yoga traces its history to the Hindu culture of India, it is not a religion.

This chapter explains the relative values of self-taught yoga, compared to attending yoga classes or seeking individual instruction. It also includes a step-by-step illustrated guide to *modified* yoga positions that are safe for people with back problems.

A few of our Back Pain Survey participants learned yoga entirely on their own, from books and articles. But those who were helped the most got started with professional and personalized instruction. Not all yoga teachers have the experience or the desire to work effectively with people who report a history of back problems. Some of them, however, possess advanced degrees in exercise physiology and may be especially qualified to prescribe exercise. An important determinant of success is the instructor's willingness to modify the therapy to suit your needs.

If yoga instruction is available where you live, we encourage you to drop by the school or studio and speak with an instructor. You may get a chance to see the instructors in action, and determine whether you feel you'll get the kind of intelligent, individual attention that you were hoping to find.

Before we extol yoga any further, however, we must interject a note of caution: Many formal yoga positions are dangerous to attempt during any episode of pain. This is especially true for just-recovering back sufferers.

At least two regular yoga positions could actually cause considerable injury to your back if you tried to perform them while you were in pain, or before you had developed the necessary flexibility. One is the Cobra, which calls for you to lie on your stomach and arch your back by raising your head and chest. The other is the Plow, in which you lie on your back, then raise your straightened legs (ouch!) up and over your head, until you can touch your toes behind your head.

Here's one yoga exercise that you can perform anywhere, as it involves nothing more than deep breathing to help you relax and tone your abdominal muscles:

- Start by taking a deep breath from your abdomen. (Put your fingers on your belly to convince yourself that it—and not just your chest—is expanding.)
- Keep inhaling through your nose for six seconds.
- Hold the air inside your lungs for three seconds.
- Exhale through your mouth for seven seconds. As you do so, let yourself go limp.
- Repeat this series of steps a few times. Five minutes spent in this kind of deep, relaxed breathing can make you feel both invigorated and relaxed. Try it during your peak work hours, and judge the effect for yourself.

The following series of yoga postures constitutes a safe taste of this form of exercise—provided that you are not in pain when you attempt them. Any or all of these can be combined with the stretching and strengthening exercises in chapters 8 and 9 to individualize or vary your daily regimen.

You may find that you want to attempt the Total Body Relaxation exercise twice a day, for the sheer stress relief it brings. As for the other exercises in this section, we suggest

157

that you begin with three repetitions of each. Once you are comfortable with that number, you can increase it by one repetition every other day until you are performing a total of ten repetitions.

TOTAL BODY RELAXATION

It may well take you several minutes to spread the feeling of relaxation throughout your body. There's no need to rush. Just enjoy the sensation of willing your body to relax. It will convince you that you can gain control over physical pain, as well as anxiety, stress, and fear.

Starting position: Lie on your back with a pillow under your knees, legs slightly apart, and arms at your sides.

Steps:
1. Let your body go limp, so that your neck, arms, and legs shift naturally into their most comfortable positions.
2. Think about relaxing your muscles, starting with your feet, ankles, and legs.
3. Concentrate on making the individual muscles and joints relax, working your way up your body to your neck and head.

Note: It may help you to tense some of your muscles slightly, prior to releasing and relaxing them. For example, first make a fist, and then let your hand go limp.

Some people find that doing this exercise in the dark is so relaxing that it actually helps them fall asleep!

SITTING SPINE STRETCH

Reaching over in this sitting posture, you will feel the stretch in your spine all the way down to your coccyx and sitting bones—and on into the hamstring muscles at the backs of your thighs. Please be careful not to push too far.

Starting position: Sit on the floor with your legs fully extended in front of you, your ankles touching each other. *a*

Steps:
1. Raise your arms in front of you to about shoulder height. *b*

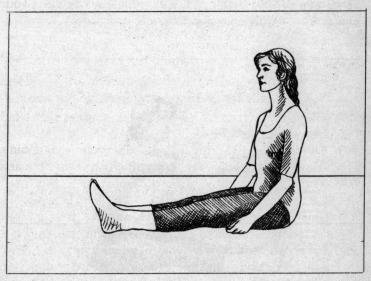

a

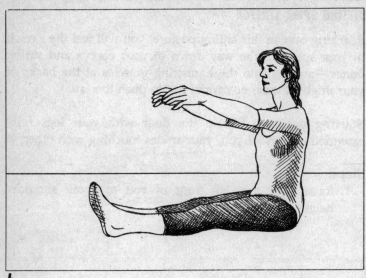

b

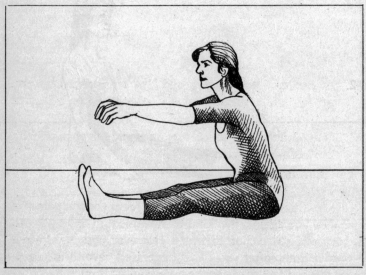

c

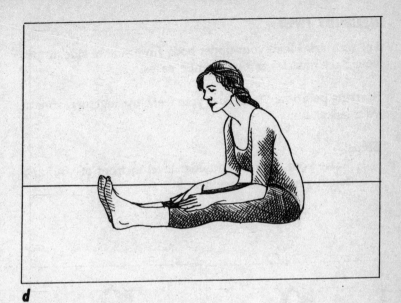

d

2. Slowly lean your upper body as far forward as you can *(c)*, while simultaneously lowering your hands to your knees. *d*
3. When you feel resistance, stop and hold the position for a count of ten.
4. Return to the starting position.

Note: This exercise is definitely not for anyone in pain. We cautioned you against this kind of movement in the note with the Hamstring Stretch in chapter 8. However, you might add it to your regimen after you have progressed beyond the pain-free stage and feel ready for more advanced stretching.

FLEXIBILITY TWIST

Let your arms lead your upper body from side to side, to put your back muscles through gentle paces.

Starting position: Stand with your feet close together, arms at your sides. *a*

Steps:

1. Raise your arms to shoulder level in front of you, and touch your hands together. *b*

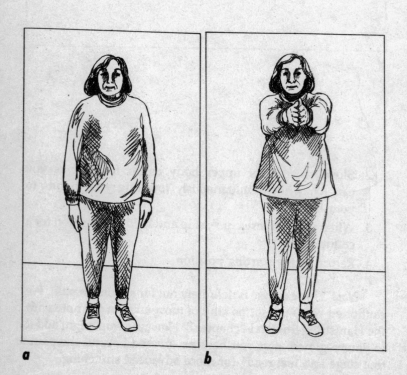

a *b*

2. Slowly turn your upper body to the left. **c**
3. When you meet resistance, hold the stretch for ten seconds. (If you find it tough to keep your balance as you twist your upper body with your feet close together, widen your stance a bit.)
4. Return to the starting position, dropping your arms and relaxing for a few seconds.
5. Repeat steps 1–4, turning to the right this time. **d**

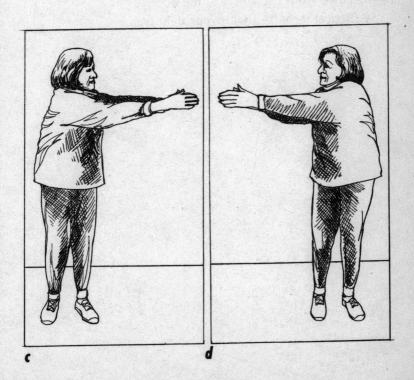

c   d

MODIFIED LOCUST

A strategically placed pillow under your abdomen keeps you from arching your back as you raise your legs in this modified locust position.

Starting position: Lie facedown, arms at your sides, with a pillow tucked under your abdomen for lower back support.

Steps:
1. Keeping your knee locked, raise your left leg about a foot off the floor. *a*
2. Hold your leg in this position for a count of six.
3. Lower your leg slowly to the floor.
4. Repeat steps 1–3 with your right leg. *b*

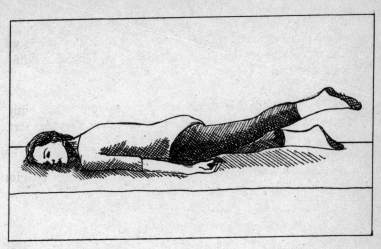

a

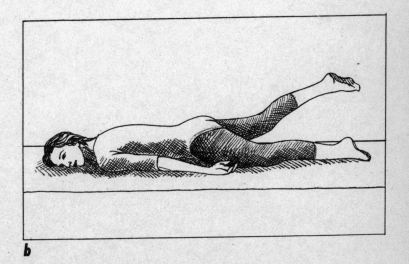

b

CHAPTER 13

Meditation, Imagery, and More

Although we don't believe that stress necessarily causes back pain, there is no doubt that incapacitating back pain causes stress. And stress, in turn, can readily magnify the pain you feel.

Certain kinds of back pain, according to reports from the participants in our Back Pain Survey, seem more susceptible to aggravation by stress than others. Neck pain, for example, tends to worsen noticeably in times of increased stress. More than 80 percent of survey participants who suffered from neck pain said their pain grew worse whenever they were under a lot of stress. A possible explanation is that stress and tension make you hunch or stiffen your shoulders, and this strain makes itself felt in the muscles of the neck.

If you have been making the rounds, seeing different practitioners over a long period of time, you may have heard the term "stress" used as though it were a diagnosis. When no obvious cause can be found for your pain, someone is bound to suggest that you are suffering from stress. Implicit in this suggestion are several negative messages, including the following:

"There's nothing really wrong with you."

"You've let stress get the upper hand in your life, and now you're paying the price."

"I can't do a thing to help you."

If stress is an element in your pain cycle, you deserve some sympathy, not blame. Doctors who understand the connection between pain and stress can help their patients greatly by explaining it—and by encouraging them to learn a few simple stress-reduction techniques that can serve as pain-blockers.

By "stress reduction" we mean reducing the negative effects of stress—the sensation that your heart is racing away, the knots in your stomach, the rapid breathing, the rising panic, the feeling of spasm in your back or neck. Whether or not you can actually reduce the stress in your life is another matter entirely. The most stressful events or situations may simply be beyond your power to control. Nevertheless, if you can control your reactions to them, you've accomplished a great deal.

Stress-reduction techniques—including deep breathing, visualization, and meditation—can be of great use in helping you feel calmer, reducing your pain, and preparing you for exercise. This chapter explains how to practice a few stress-reduction techniques to best advantage. Think of them as mental exercises, easy and pleasant to perform.

The truth is, any technique that provides a break from

stressful activities may turn out to help your back. Even something as simple as taking a "stretch break" every hour on the hour can be of tremendous benefit. Although we urge you to experiment with the proven effective strategies of deep breathing, meditation, visualization (or imagery), and progressive relaxation, we know of many people who can get their stress *and* pain levels down by taking a walk for twenty minutes.

Our survey participants, as a group, came up with no clear consensus on a favorite method, but individuals expressed strong preferences. Many vendors of relaxation tapes and stress-reduction gadgets may try to convince you that their approach is the best, but you are the best judge of what technique appeals to you most, and therefore what is most likely to work for you.

Practitioners of yoga know that deep breathing has tremendous powers of relaxation. Just as smiling can sometimes lift your spirits, breathing slowly and deeply can make your whole body feel calmer. Deep breathing figures in virtually every stress-reduction technique, so we'll begin with this basic approach.

Deep Breathing

Ordinarily, you don't have to think about breathing. Your body does it automatically. But when the automatic response is panting in response to some stress perceived as a threat, you can make yourself feel better by taking conscious control of the breathing process. Try it. Inhale through your nose for six seconds; hold your breath for one second; exhale through your mouth for seven seconds. Keep your eyes closed. Do you feel yourself getting a bit more relaxed with each exhalation?

Try to become conscious of the breath filling and leaving your lungs. Let your chest expand fully. Relax your shoulders as you inhale, since raising your shoulders does not help to fill the lungs with air. Concentrate instead on widening the girth of your chest, as though it were a balloon being inflated. Put your hand on your abdomen, to feel how it, too, is expanding, as your diaphragm drops down to increase the influx of air into your body.

Stay relaxed as you hold the air in for just a moment or two, and then slowly begin to let it out through your mouth. Exhale so fully that you actually squeeze the air out of your lungs by contracting your chest. Then picture physical tension leaving your body with the expelled breath.

Once you become accustomed to deep breathing, knowing that you can rely on it as an instant aid to relaxation, you may find that you use it periodically throughout the day, any time something unpleasant jars you. You may also use deep breathing at night as a way to relax before falling asleep, and again in the morning, to prepare yourself to meet the day.

Meditation

Heart specialists such as Dr. Herbert Benson of Harvard Medical School and Dr. Dean Ornish of the Preventive Medicine Research Institute in Sausalito, California, have made meditation a medical treatment. Back sufferers benefit from its stress-reducing effects, too. It was Dr. Benson who gave the name "relaxation response" to the altered state of well-being brought on by meditation. The relaxation response is a physiological state of deep rest while wide awake. It is said to be even more restful and restorative than sleep, because the profound relaxation leaves a lingering sense of calm refreshment. Indeed, a twenty-minute period of meditation may exert a positive effect on an entire day.

Many approaches to meditation can be used to good advantage, but we particularly like Dr. Benson's approach.

The basic outline here is drawn from his book called *Your Maximum Mind*:

- Choose a word or a phrase that will serve as your focus for the meditation exercise. You may choose a pleasant thought, such as "peace," or the opening words of a prayer, or even a soothing sound that has no particular meaning.
- Sit in a comfortable position. Close your eyes. Relax your muscles.
- Breathe deeply and, with each exhalation, repeat to yourself your focus word or phrase.
- Also use the repetition of your focus word to push away worries or extraneous thoughts that may come into your mind while you are meditating.
- Continue your focused breathing and repetition for ten to twenty minutes.

It sounds awfully simple, doesn't it? But please don't let the simplicity fool you into thinking that there's nothing much to it. Practice brings total concentration, and total concentration breeds relaxation that works to reduce stress and improve the quality of your life.

If possible, choose a special place for meditation. You might even keep a few items there—photos or memorabilia—that evoke positive feelings. Also try to choose a special time of day when you are least likely to be interrupted. Avoid distractions by taking your phone off the hook, or by asking family and friends not to call you at this time.

Visualization (Imagery)

The power of positive thinking makes it possible for you to soothe yourself with beautiful images that you conjure up and elaborate upon in your mind. These could be landscapes, works of art, or wonderful moments in your life. The idea of visualization is to create a safe haven in your mind where you can go to escape from pain or anxiety.

If this sounds farfetched, try to remember a time when you had the opposite experience—when thinking of a sad event left you feeling depressed, or when planning what you would say in an argument got you so worked up you could barely sit still. The brain and body seem to make little distinction between actual images and imagined ones. This is why you can create the sensation of peaceful relaxation by picturing an idyllic scene where you lie on warm sand, smelling the salt air of the ocean, and hearing the waves pounding on the shore.

Another positive image is to picture a soft glove or gentle hand touching the painful areas of your body with warmth and healing power.

Progressive Relaxation

Relaxing your body inch by inch, one small part at a time, gets you progressively relaxed until you reach the critical threshold where stress-reduction occurs.

Progressive Relaxation resembles the Total Body Relaxation described in chapter 12. The idea here is to get relaxed by first tensing the muscles and then releasing them, proceeding in an orderly fashion from one end of the body to the other. It doesn't really matter whether you go from head to toe or begin at your feet and work up.

Here is a plan of action:

- Lie in a comfortable position. Close your eyes.
- Move your body, wriggling your arms and legs, just to settle yourself comfortably.
- Lie still and breathe deeply for a few minutes.

- If you are starting from your head, make some very exaggerated movements with your face—sneer, grin, frown, yawn, raise your eyebrows and then knit them together in a scowl. Then let your face relax.
- Tense your neck by lifting your head, then lie back.
- One at a time, tighten each arm and raise it, then let it go limp at your side.
- Clench each fist, then let your hands relax.
- Tighten your abdomen and your buttocks, and let them go.
- Spread tension along the length of one leg by straightening the knee and lifting the leg slightly. Then relax that leg and let it slump back into place. Do the same with your other leg.
- Point your toes and arch your foot as sharply as you can, then let it flop free. Do the same with your other foot.
- Lie still and breathe deeply.

You may find that you want to experiment with the different approaches, or mix and match them. What's to stop you, for example, from using a favorite image as your meditation focus?

As you become adept at incorporating these stress-reduction techniques into your daily routines, people may ask you why you're smiling.

P A R T
F I V E

Lifestyle Changes

> Small adjustments in performing everyday activities count among the most important steps toward achieving freedom from back pain.

CHAPTER 14

Positioning Yourself

The chair you sit in, the mattress you sleep on, the posture you assume while sitting or standing—all these factors collectively influence the amount of back pain you suffer. Our Back Pain Survey participants found that they could increase their comfort throughout the day by choosing the best positions for all activities—and that includes inactivity, too.

The idea of this careful, close scrutiny may seem daunting at first. If you have to police yourself all the time, how can you ever relax and enjoy life? You can, because once you get the basic idea of keeping your back in a relaxed yet correct posture, you will begin to feel the benefits of doing so. You'll have less pain, and be able to do more. As practice becomes habit, you won't have to think continually about how you're standing or holding your head. By then, all these good measures will have become second nature to you.

In this chapter, we offer numerous suggestions that we hope will help you move through the day with the greatest of ease. Let's start first thing in the morning, with the moment you get out of bed.

Getting Out of Bed

Many people who wouldn't attempt a sit-up on a bet actually try to pull themselves out of bed with their abdominal muscles. We want you to exercise, of course, but only when you're warmed up and ready. Getting out of bed need not be an exercise challenge.

To make the process easy on yourself, ease your way over to the side of the bed, so that you are lying on your side with your knees bent, facing the edge. If you choose to lie on your left side, then you can place your right palm on the mattress next to your left shoulder. In one fluid motion, push down with your right palm and swing yourself upright, taking your legs off the bed and setting your feet on the floor. Now, keeping your back straight, stand up. If you like, you can use both hands to push yourself to a standing position.

Washing Up

When you brush your teeth or wash your face at the bathroom sink, you needn't stand at attention. Try keeping your back straight and bending your knees just a bit. This precaution takes the strain off your hamstrings when you lean forward to splash water on your face.

Standing

Try to pay constant attention to your posture. Keep your abdomen, buttocks, and chin tucked in, and the rest of your body will tend to follow suit and line up properly. Your abdominal muscles, which hold in your gut, give the all-important support to your lower back when they are in this tucked-in position. Tucking in your buttocks, which naturally fits with pulling in your abdominals, helps normalize the S-shaped curve in your lower back, and thereby ease pain. Tucking in your chin helps you maintain the proper curve in your neck, easing the strain on that part of your spine.

We simply can't overemphasize the importance of good posture as a way to hasten recovery from acute episodes of low-back pain, and to prevent future episodes from occurring.

Good posture does not require you to distribute your weight evenly on both legs at all times. If you need to stand in one place for a spell, as in a ticket line or a checkout line, for example, try shifting your weight from one foot to the other every few minutes. In other situations where you need to be on your feet for extended periods, the best way to pass the time may be to walk about instead of standing rooted to the spot.

Sitting

More important than the chair you sit in is the time you spend sitting. Since sitting offers more opportunity for back aggravation than either standing or lying down, you may need to limit your sitting time. Whenever possible, break up long sits by getting up to stretch. You can do this most easily at home, of course, but try to stretch at work, too. If you're driving on a long car trip, let yourself stop frequently for stretch breaks. On long plane flights, too, look for times when you can move about in the aisles, and seize the opportunity.

Good sitting posture means planting yourself firmly on your bottom, with your abdominals pulled in to help keep your lower back straight. Common sitting habits that could cause you grief include slouching back in your chair, leaning too far forward, and crossing your legs. Instead, try resting your feet on a footstool, as a way to help you sit tall and keep pressure off the backs of your thighs. (At work, some of our survey participants said they liked to open a bottom desk drawer and prop their feet on it while typing, writing, or talking on the telephone.)

Your chair owes you a firm support, both under your bottom and behind your back. If your chair isn't up to the task, you can correct it with a firm bottom support or a back-support cushion, or both, so as to avoid any strain or discomfort. Many varieties of firm chair pads and backrests, including some models that combine both types of support, are sold in stores and by mail order. Try to experiment to find one that feels right for you—and is priced right, too.

If you love to attend outdoor concerts or sporting events where you're expected to sit on backless bleachers, you may want to invest in a stadium chair—a padded seat and back support that clamps right onto the bleachers.*

Holding Your Own

In general, we found that our survey participants did best when they held their postures by the strength of their own muscles, instead of relying on back braces and cervical collars. Although these devices seem designed to be helpful, they can actually keep you from developing the good habit of good

*Bleachers = benches

posture. What's more, immobilizing any part of your body is almost always a poor alternative to exercising it gently and moving it correctly.

Talking on the Telephone

You can easily talk yourself into a pain in the neck with a telephone. The temptation to free your hands by cradling the phone between your shoulder and your ear (and leaving it there indefinitely) is almost irresistible. Phone rests that encourage this behavior were definitely *not* designed for people who suffer from neck or back pain. If you must have your hands free while you carry on telephone conversations, by all means invest in a speakerphone or a headset that gives you mobility without muscle strain.

Working

Depending on the demands your job makes on your back, you may find that you need to make some adjustments at your workplace. A few offices and industries now offer on-the-job education programs aimed specifically at showing employees how to avoid back injuries. We applaud these efforts, and expect to see more of them.

If you have a regular office job, it may be possible for you to accomplish the same amount of work in a new position. Several of our survey participants, in fact, reported that they could work more effectively on their feet. A few of them were allowed to add height to their desks by setting up a crate or lectern on the desk surface, which allowed them to do their deskwork standing up.

If your job calls for a lot of typing into a computer, try to arrange your workstation so that you can comfortably read what you need to type. Copy holders that attach to the side of the computer monitor, at eye level, can help you avoid neck and back strain.

Taking Breaks

Even if you maintain ideal posture sitting and standing, you can go yourself one better by taking a few respites, of just five to ten minutes each, every day. During these breaks, try to put yourself in a completely different position. One of the most popular among our survey participants was lying on the floor with feet and calves propped up on a sofa or chair, for ten minutes at a time.

The strain-easing posture can also prove to be a break from stress if you spend this time engaged in deep breathing.

Reading and Watching Television

Try to catch up on your reading *before* bedtime, so you can hold a book at a comfortable eye level on a table or desk. If you like to sit in a special armchair that won't tuck under a table, then pile some pillows in your lap to help support the book, rather than tilting your neck down and straining to see it.

If you regularly read in bed by placing a couple of pillows under your head to help you see the book or magazine propped on your abdomen, you have probably noticed that this position soon produces neck strain or eyestrain or both. And if you hold your reading material over your head while you're lying down, you strain your shoulders, neck, and back. Indeed, most of our survey participants reported, with some remorse, that reading in bed was one pastime they had to learn to live without. They substituted reading just before retiring—sitting up in a good chair, or standing, with the book propped up on a box atop a kitchen counter.

Television viewing, too, is best done from a chair—if you want to keep your neck happy. But since you don't have to hold the television(!), it's easier to watch TV while lying down than to read in that position. Try to assume a position that would be comfortable for sleeping, such as lying on your side, with a pillow under your head and neck.

Driving

You'll probably find that sitting in a car can be made more manageable with a back support of some kind. Our survey participants particularly liked car seats or back cushions that aligned their backs at a right angle to their thighs, which provided maximum driving comfort.

Other positioning strategies that help are pulling the driver's seat as close as possible to the steering wheel. This closeness will enable you to sit with your knees slightly elevated, and to diminish the strain that often comes from overreaching to reach the wheel. You can also make use of the built-in armrest on the left-hand door for added arm support. And if you drive a car with bucket seats, you may have a divider or equipment box at your right that doubles as a second armrest.

When you get in or out of a car, try to eliminate awkward leg stretches and body twists. For example, on entering the vehicle, open the door and then turn your back to the seat, so you can sit straight down. Then bring in your legs, using your abdominal muscles for support, and turn to face forward. Similarly, when getting out of the car, move yourself to the very edge of the seat, turn sideways, and then put your feet on the ground and stand up.

Getting into Bed

Back up to your bed until you can feel it with the backs of your legs, so you won't be tempted to twist or turn around to see where you're going. Pull in your abdominal muscles to keep your back straight, and sit down. Then, reversing the fluid motion that got you out of bed this morning, and using your arms and hands to help support and guide your body, lie down on your side as you swing your legs onto the bed.

Now that you're in bed, and given the fact that you spend one-third of your life in it, how happy are you with your mattress? Most people with back pain find that even a firm mattress feels better if it's positioned on top of a three-quarter-inch-thick plywood bedboard. On the road, many of our survey participants carry folding bedboards that can fit into a suitcase, just in case the bed at the hotel or motel where they're heading doesn't stack up to the comfort of their own beds.

Positions for Lovemaking

Our survey participants spoke candidly about positions that enabled them to make love without making trouble for their backs. The most frequently recommended position called for both partners to lie on their sides, with knees bent, facing each other. Lying front to back, nested like spoons, with the man behind the woman, is another safe position for sexual intercourse. If you are comfortable lying on your back with your knees elevated—and if your partner is strong enough to keep most of his or her weight off you—then this modified missionary position is also a safe one.

We heard the three suggestions listed above repeatedly from survey participants who said they had an active sex life despite back pain. Others declined to mention specific positions, but stressed the importance of maintaining open communication with one's partner—and openness to sexual pleasures other than intercourse.

Sleeping

Most people with low-back pain find that the most comfortable way to sleep is on one's side, in a modified fetal position. Try it, keeping your pillow tucked under your head and neck only, and not under your shoulders. A relatively flat pillow seems to work better than a very fluffy one, because it won't raise your head so high as to strain your neck. To further reduce any strain on your spine, try putting a thin pillow between your knees.

If you have neck pain, you may find that your most comfortable sleep position is on your back, with one pillow under your head and neck, and another one or two pillows propped under your knees, to keep your back from arching.

Sleeping on the stomach (a position many people love) is, sad to say, the toughest on the back. If you cannot break this habit, no matter how hard you try, then at least try to do without a pillow under your head. Put the pillow under your tummy instead—to minimize the arching of your back.

CHAPTER 15

Accomplishing Tasks

Doing what needs to be done—that's just what people with back pain too often find they can't do. Or they're afraid to do those things, for fear of creating more back trouble. Yet a few simple precautions can help anyone perform everyday activities without pain or risk of injury, and many inventive gadgets can make any number of jobs easier to tackle. These kinds of moment-to-moment strategies, many of them drawn from our Back Pain Survey participants' experiences, add up to a back-friendly lifestyle.

In addition to our survey results on the importance of approaching tasks in ways that make good back sense, medical doctors have also endorsed such measures. The prestigious

Quebec Task Force, a group of doctors reviewing back treatments, found that the two most important means of improving back fitness are exercise and learning how to safeguard your back as you go about doing what you have to do—and doing what you love to do—at work, at home, and on the road.

This chapter takes the back into account while analyzing everyday activities from bathing to housework and yard work. It describes ways of doing chores, as well as techniques for lifting and carrying that can help you avoid painful backache.

Lifting

Every time you pick up an object from the floor, whether it's a pin or a bag of groceries, you have the opportunity to hurt your back—or help it. The participants in our Back Pain Survey waxed eloquent on the topic of lifting. In fact, they were downright adamant about bending at the knees—not at the waist—to pick up *anything*, whether it's as light as a tissue or as heavy as a potted plant. Bending at the knees allows you to keep your back straight as you stoop, and to take the weight of whatever you're lifting with your legs instead of your back.

If you find it difficult to squat in this fashion, or to stand up again after you do, you can try placing a chair or stepladder near you for support.

To further minimize any risk of injury, hold the item you're lifting close to your body. This is especially important with heavy items. And speaking of heavy items, always ask yourself first if you really need to lift them. Maybe you can slide them to their destination, or enlist someone else's aid.

Another approach to heavy lifting, although it sounds awkward, is to turn your back to the object and extend your arms *behind* you. When in doubt, ask for help.

Carrying

Less is preferable to more in this department. Try to lighten the load of your shoulder bag, pocketbook, or briefcase. You might even consider using a backpack instead. Although it looks less elegant, it distributes weight more evenly and often proves to be the most comfortable way to transport everyday items.

When you buy your groceries, pack them in two bags of equal weight, with carrying handles. It is much easier to carry groceries with your arms at your sides than to clutch bags to your chest or balance them on your hips. Lifting your arms while holding heavy packages puts more strain on the back, participants say. Better yet, consider buying a wheeled shopping cart for bringing home large orders—or see if your supermarket will deliver them.

Child Care

The least stressful way to carry an infant a long distance is on your back in a carrier. The hip carry, in comparison, caused pain for most of our survey participants who had young children.

If your baby and your back act up at the same time, try holding or comforting your child while you kneel at his or her level—or while both of you are lying down. Another favorite position is to sit in a rocking chair while feeding or lulling an infant to sleep.

Be advised that most of the furniture designed for babies —bassinets, playpens, even cribs—can play havoc with a parent's back. They all involve leaning at awkward angles, whether you are putting your child in them or taking him out. If your child is sleeping in a crib, drop the collapsible side before you reach in, so you can bend at your knees instead of leaning over the bars. Take the same approach to the child's playpen.

Some of our participants replaced the bassinet with a large wicker laundry basket, lined with soft blankets and set on the floor.

A notable exception in this back-straining category is the adjustable changing table, which can be raised to the right height for your back, allowing you to diaper and dress your baby in comfort.

Making Your Bed

As with any job that requires you to lower yourself, bend at your knees instead of at your waist. You can stay in a kneeling position as you work your way around the bed. Go slowly, and reposition yourself as often as necessary to avoid overstretching your back.

Unless your bed rolls easily, you'll do best to keep it at least a foot away from the wall, so that you can smooth the sheets and blankets from all sides with equal effort.

If you're in pain, let yourself off the hook and don't bother making the bed at all.

Getting Organized

Standing on tiptoe and reaching to retrieve boxes and jars from high shelves can aggravate back pain. Try to save yourself a certain amount of reaching high overhead and stooping to the floor by organizing your cupboards and closets with your back in mind. For example, instead of parking your shoes on the closet floor, hang them in a shoebag on the door.

In any storage area, try to put the things you use most

often at the most convenient height. For getting to those infrequently used items that live on high shelves, keep a sturdy stepladder handy.

Washing Dishes

Leaning over the sink to wash dishes may cause problems for your back. Automatic dishwashers don't necessarily solve these problems, since loading and unloading them may make even more demands on your back than washing the old-fashioned way.

You can ease the reach across to the faucets by turning sideways. It's usually easier to reach sideways than forward. Once the water is running, stand close to the sink for minimal strain. Belly up to it, in fact, and use a waterproof apron to keep yourself dry.

As you wash individual items, lift them out of the sink and hold them close, too. Shift your weight from one foot to the other on long stints. Or simply place one foot on a footstool to help keep your back relaxed. And do break up the task by letting pots and pans soak awhile. You can always go back to them later.

Vacuuming

Judging from comments offered by our survey participants, the people who suffer the most back pain from vacuuming are those who strive for perfection in this chore. The best advice seems to be to lower your standards a bit, and don't feel guilty about leaving some dust if that means sparing your back.

Maneuver the machine with one hand, and leave the other at your side. Fifteen minutes at a time makes a reasonable round of vacuuming. But by all means stop before that if you feel the fatigue in your back.

Please don't vacuum when you're in pain, no matter who is coming to dinner.

If you're in the market for a new vacuum cleaner, look for one that you can push with minimal exertion.

Other Household Chores

For mopping, choose a sponge mop that you can wring out from the far end of the handle, with no leaning over. These are readily available in supermarkets and hardware stores. You may find that you can stand up straighter if you hold the mop with one hand instead of two.

Whenever and wherever possible, extend your reach with long-handled gadgets that do the reaching for you, and enable you to keep your own arms and hands close to your sides. Shops and mail-order catalogs carry specially made items that will help you pick items from shelves or off the floor, scrub the bathtub without stretching across it, and wash windows from a safe vantage point. There's even a dustpan and brush with handles long enough to let you collect your sweepings while standing tall.

There are a number of organizations in the UK which supply equipment and back-friendly house cleaning tools for those who have difficulty in using 'ordinary' equivalents. A list of names and addresses, including companies that offer a mail order service, is given under 'Helpful Addresses' on page 201.

Painting

If you feel up to tackling a big chore like this one, good for you! Make it a safe-back activity by standing as close as you possibly can to whatever you're painting. This will allow you to strike the best posture and keep your arms close to your body for minimal back strain. Also try to position yourself so that you need not raise your arms higher than your chest or lower than past your waist.

Choose your weapon with an eye to getting the job done quickly and easily. Rollers work best because they are light and efficient. Paintbrushes take longer, and paint guns, though fast, are heavy to hold for any appreciable time.

Pace yourself, as you would on any big project. Remember that it makes no sense to finish the job the day you start it—if doing so threatens to finish you.

If you insist on painting the ceilings yourself, protect your neck by looking down frequently. Treat yourself to a one-minute break every five minutes and a ten-minute break every half hour. By all means, do the neck and shoulder exercises described in chapter 9.

Raking Leaves

Autumn leaves, like winter snows, probably cause several million Americans to seek professional treatment for back pain every year. Please keep yourself out of these grim statistics by approaching seasonal chores with extra caution.

The danger lies in excessive forward leaning and arm extension. These awkward, unsupported positions leave your back vulnerable to injury.

When you rake, keep your knees in the unlocked, or slightly bent, position. When it's time to pick up the leaves you've raked into piles, kneel or squat rather than stooping. To carry bags of leaves safely, take two small bags of equal weight at a time, with your arms at your sides. Holding a large bag out in front of your body can readily harm your back.

Many special tools can make this job easier, including a rake with a bend in the handle that allows you to stand up straighter as you work, shifting a greater share of the effort from your back to your arms. Another back-saver is a large-wheeled garden cart (not a wheelbarrow) that lets you wheel your leaves to the curb.

Shoveling Snow

Do dress yourself in layers before tackling this task, so you can keep your back warm throughout, but shed clothing as the effort of shoveling heats your body.

When hefting the shovel, remember to bend your legs and not your back. Keep the shovel as close to your body as you can, and keep the size of each shovelful modest. Wet snow makes for heavy lifting.

Gardening

Although it is theoretically possible to work in your garden without bending at the waist or working your back into a state of fatigue, few people do. They'd just as soon try to keep their hands clean while working the soil. The effort seems to come between them and the basic joy of gardening. A solution offered by one of our survey participants was to lie down on her side to pull weeds.

When people ask you what gifts you'd like for your birthday or other occasion, give them the names of garden tools designed for people with back problems. These include tongs that scoop up piles of leaves and weeds, long-handled tools, lightweight hoses on retractable reels, and connectors that allow easy access to hard-to-reach outdoor spigots.

C H A P T E R 16

Enjoying Life

As you stretch and strengthen your back with the helpful exercises you've learned, you will grow increasingly more flexible and resistant to future back injury. This is a great gift that you are giving yourself—one that will enable you to enjoy life more fully.

When we reviewed the comments of survey participants who had resolved years or even decades of chronic back pain, we noticed another "gift" of theirs. It was nothing as tangible as an exercise program or a set of strategies for completing chores. It was their attitude.

They had promised themselves that they would get well. They had made up their minds to put an end to back pain.

And they had put themselves in charge of that task, giving it top priority in their lives. They had stopped asking "Why me?" They had come to accept their back problem, and that acceptance was the key to finding a solution.

Realizing that they knew more about their own bodies than anyone else possibly could, they listened to the experts without awe. They sought professional care when they needed to, but they did not expect any practitioner to have "the answer" or to "cure" them. They acted as partners in their treatment. Even though they were suffering, they did not see themselves as helpless victims waiting to be rescued by someone else.

Exercise can help you develop this attitude of mastery. Exercise is a powerful, effective treatment that you dispense to yourself on a daily basis. In a relatively short time, you can see it working as promised, building your body and your confidence at the same time.

As you improve your ability to enjoy life by treating your body with exercise, you will be disproving some long-standing myths about back pain. Maybe you've heard some of these myths, or believed in them yourself:

• *Back pain is inevitable. It's just the price we pay for walking upright.* Pain is not the natural condition of the body. If anything, back pain results from not walking upright enough. Although back pain is extremely common in the United States, where it affects an estimated 80 percent of all adults, statistics from other countries indicate a much lower incidence. Back pain, therefore, is not an essential part of the human condition, but a reflection of lifestyle trends. We in the United States have adopted an excessively sedentary lifestyle. But that can be changed at will. Exercise, coupled with attention to posture and care in performing daily tasks, will convince your body that there is nothing inevitable about back pain.

• *Back pain is a normal aspect of aging.* Again, pain is neither natural nor normal. Aging does not hurt, unless it is accompanied by illness or neglect of one's health. Analyses of national medical records show that back pain is *not* correlated with advanced age. In fact, the reverse is true: The vast majority of backache sufferers are younger than forty-five. As you grow older, treating your body well, you have every reason to expect that your back pain will continue to diminish until it disappears altogether.

• *There's nothing really wrong with you.* Even if nothing shows up on the X rays or other diagnostic tests, even if the doctor cannot imagine why you are in pain, there *is* something really wrong with you if you are in pain.

• *Any exercise program will help banish back pain.* This is only half true. You know, if you've tried exercise before, that not all routines work for all people. Some noninjurious exercise is better than no exercise, but an individually prescribed program, or the tailored program you have now assembled from the ingredients offered here, can do much more for you than can an "off-the-rack" exercise regimen. (Indeed, we remind you that strenuous, arching forms of exercise can wreck backs.)

• *Back practitioners routinely offer exercise advice, but back sufferers are too lazy to follow it.* You know from your own experience just how much exercise advice you were offered. Maybe it was an encouraging word, with a few specific suggestions, but more likely you came to the exercise conclusion yourself. You've turned to this book for detailed instructions about assembling and implementing an exercise program. And now you're going to stick to that program because you want to improve your own condition. You are taking action, and you will succeed.

Many of the participants in our Back Pain Survey expressed the opinion that their *approach* to back exercise—and

by that they meant their attitude and preparation for exercise
—was at least as important as the mechanical components of
the exercise therapy itself. Here are some points to remember
as you implement your exercise program over the coming
weeks:

• Exercise therapy is more beneficial for your back than
anything you can put into or onto your body.
• Although your exercise movements may be slow and
gradual now, they will result in dramatic improvements over
time. You can expect small but noticeable gains within a few
weeks.
• If exercise is something you've never looked forward to
before, open your mind to enjoying it now. The time you
spend exercising truly is quality time.

As you become used to exercising, you may wonder how
you ever got along without it. When you miss a few days of
walking or swimming or cycling, you'll miss the relaxation
and clear thinking that those activities convey. You'll miss the
reassuring physical sensation of tiredness followed by re-
newed energy. These are the positive additions to your life
that exercise has brought. You will be eager to get back to
exercising to experience again these pleasant feelings. Exercise, which you once may have viewed as a duty, is now a
delight for you—an indulgence of body and mind that you
enjoy thoroughly.

To add to your enjoyment of exercise and your new
feeling of vitality, try some of the following physical rewards
as treats for your body:

• *Massage.* Like exercise, massage offers you another drug-
free muscle relaxant that will help your muscles unwind. You
can perform self-massage on some areas of your body, but you
will probably get the most pleasure out of a full-body massage

from a professional—or even from a willing partner. You may need to tell your inexperienced masseur to use a light oil and a fairly light touch, so as to avoid putting too much pressure on your lower back. Also tell your partner to concentrate on your legs, back, and neck, massaging toward the heart, and using either a long, gliding motion with the palms, or a circular motion with the fingertips and palms.

• *Good food.* Feeding your body well is part of pampering yourself. Try to eat more fruits, vegetables, and whole grains, and to cut down on junk foods, processed foods, fats, caffeine, sugar, and alcohol. Also, avoid constipation (a real hardship for back sufferers) by drinking enough water and including generous portions of fiber in your diet. You may notice a positive change in the appearance of your body, brought on by your commitment to exercise and good posture. Taking care to eat only good foods will help you keep your weight in the ideal range for your height, so that you look even better.

• *Sleep.* Promise yourself the amount of sleep you need to feel comfortable and to maintain good spirits and good posture throughout the day. Try not to think of time spent sleeping as lost or wasted. It isn't. It's crucial time spent restoring your mental and physical energy.

• *Hydrotherapy.* Turn your tub into a relaxing hydrotherapy center where you can enjoy luxurious warm baths. You may want to purchase a waterproof pillow or a mat that covers the full length of your tub. A less expensive alternative is to pad the tub bottom with a thick bath mat, and roll a towel into a neck support or a lumbar support. Our survey participants consider twenty minutes the ideal length for a bath, as longer can make you feel tired. They also prefer warm water to hot, since very hot water can sometimes put muscles in spasm. Experiment to find the most comfortable position. A safe one is to lean your back against one end of the tub, and bend your knees so you can keep your feet flat on the bottom of the tub. If you feel stiff after maintaining one position for several minutes, prop your feet on the sides of the tub for a change. You can even execute a few exercises in the tub, such as shoulder shrugs and knee-to-chest stretches.

• *Join a health club.* Although you can perform all your exercises perfectly well right at home, you may still benefit from joining a local health club. If, for example, the club has a swimming pool and a whirlpool that you can use, these facilities may be worth the price of membership. You can take advantage of the swimming pool for aerobic fitness, and the whirlpool for relaxation and stress reduction. Membership in a health club also puts you in touch with other people who are trying to keep their bodies in the best possible shape, just as you are.

You are about to join the ranks of back sufferers who have beaten the rap—who have endured the pain and gotten past it. You have decided what you need to do to get well, and you are putting that plan into effect right now.

We salute you in your efforts.

RECOMMENDED READING

The following books may be of some further help to you. If you find that any of the titles are out of print, you should be able to find them in your local library.

Campbell, Dr Anthony   *Getting the Best for Your Bad Back* Sheldon Press 1992.

Imrie, David and Simson Coleen   *Goodbye Backache: A New Approach in Three Steps towards the Prevention and Treatment of Backache* Sheldon Press 1984.

Madders, Jane   *Stress and Relaxation* Positive Health Guides.

Stoddard, Dr Alan   *The Back: Relief from Pain* Optime 1990.

Tanner, Dr J.   *Beating Back Pain* Dorling Kindersley 1987.

The Which Guide to Managing Back Trouble Which? 1996.

HELPFUL ADDRESSES

The following list of addresses includes some self-help organizations for back pain sufferers, as well as a number of complementary and alternative practitioners' associations from whom you can get a list of registered therapists in your area.

Arthritis and Rheumatism Council
   17 Cleland Park South, Bangor, County Down, Northern Ireland BT20 3EW. Tel.: 01247 463109
British Chiropractic Association
   29 Whitley Street, Reading, Berkshire RG2 0EG. Tel.: 01734 757557
British Institute of Muscularskeletal Medicine
   27 Green Lane, Northwood, Middlesex HA6 2PX. Tel.: 01923 825583
The Chartered Society of Physiotherapy
   14 Bedford Row, London WC1R 4ED. Tel.: 0171 242 1941
General Council and Register of Osteopaths
   56 London Street, Reading, Berkshire RG1 4SQ. Tel.: 01734 576585
National Ankylosing Spondylitis Society
   5 Grosvenor Crescent, London SW1X 7ER. Tel.: 0171 235 9585

National Back Pain Association
   31/33 Park Road, Teddington, Middlesex TW11 0AB. Tel.: 0181 977
   5474
National Osteoporosis Society
   P O Box 10, Radstock, Bath BA3 3YB. Tel.: 01761 471771
Relaxation for Living
   168/170 Oatlands Drive, Weybridge, Surrey KT13 9ET. Tel.: 01932
   858355
Royal Association for Disability and Rehabilitation (RADAR)
   25 Mortimer Street, London W1N 8AB. Tel.: 0171 637 5400
   (Remap, which you can contact through RADAR, designs and makes
   equipment for disabled people to help them in employment.
Scoliosis Association UK
   2 Ivebury Court, 325 Latimer Road, London W10 6RA.
Scottish Chiropractic Association
   30 Roseburn Place, Edinburgh EH12 5NX. Tel.: 0131 346 7500
Self-Help in Pain (SHIP)
   33 Kingsdown Park, Tankerton, Kent CT5 2DT. Tel.: 01227 264677
Special Gymnastics Association
   Wingate House, Wrenbury Hall Drive, Wrenbury, Nr Nantwich,
   Cheshire CW5 8ES. Tel.: 01270 780456. (Exercises for all those with
   special needs.)

The following organizations supply equipment and back-friendly house cleaning tools:

The Back Shop
   24 New Cavendish Street, London W1M 7LH. Tel.: 0171 935 9148
Cape Ability
   52 St Isan Road, Heath Cardiff CF4 4LY. Tel.@ 01222 620261 (Aids for
   the elderly and disabled.)
The Keep Able Centre
   2 Capital Interchange Way, Brentford Middlesex TW8 0EX. Tel.: 0181
   7422181
Mobility Wales
   4 High Street, Cowbridge, South Glamorgan CF7 7AG. Tel.: 01446
   773393/4 (Provides mobility aids; postal service.)
Nottingham Rehab
   17 Ludlow Hill Road, West Bridgford, Nottingham NG2 6HD. Tel.:
   0115 9360319 (Mail order company.)